DEC - 2 2002

Healing
Meditation

Delmar Publishers' Online Services

To access Delmar on the World Wide Web, point your browser to:

http://www.delmar.com/delmar.html

To access through Gopher: gopher://gopher.delmar.com

(Delmar Online is part of "thomson.com", an Internet site with information on more than 30 publishers of the International Thomson Publishing organization.)

For information on our products and services:

email: info@delmar.com

or call: 800-347-7707

Healing Meditation

MARY GRACE UMLAUF, PhD, RN
Associate Professor
Graduate Program
The University of Alabama at Birmingham
Birmingham, Alabama

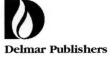

Delmar Publishers

An International Thomson Publishing Company

Albany • Bonn • Boston • Cincinnati • Detroit • London
Madrid • Melbourne • Mexico City • New York • Pacific Grove
Paris • San Francisco • Singapore • Tokyo • Toronto • Washington

NOTICE TO THE READER

Cover Design: Spiral Design
Cover Illustration: Kirsten Soderlind

Delmar Staff

Senior Acquisitions Editor: Bill Burgower
Assistant Editor: Hilary A. Schrauf
Senior Project Editor: Judith Boyd Nelson
Production Coordinator: Barbara A. Bullock
Art and Design Coordinator: Carole D. Keohane

COPYRIGHT © 1997
By Delmar Publishers
a division of International Thomson Publishing Inc.

The ITP logo is a trademark under license.

Printed in the United States of America

For more information, contact:

Delmar Publishers
3 Columbia Circle, Box 15015
Albany, New York 12212-5015

International Thomson Publishing Europe
Berkshire House 168-173
High Holborn
London, WC1V 7AA
England

Thomas Nelson Australia
102 Dodds Street
South Melbourne, 3205
Victoria, Australia

Nelson Canada
1120 Birchmount Road
Scarborough, Ontario
Canada, M1K 5G4

International Thomson Editores
Campos Eliseos 385, Piso 7
Col Polanco
11560 Mexico D F Mexico

International Thomson Publishing GmbH
Konigswinterer Strasse 418
53227 Bonn
Germany

International Thomson Publishing Asia
221 Henderson Road
#05-10 Henderson Building
Singapore 0315

International Thomson Publishing—Japan
Hirakawacho Kyowa Building, 3F
2-2-1 Hirakawacho
Chiyoda-ku, Tokyo 102
Japan

1 2 3 4 5 6 7 8 9 10 XXX 02 01 00 99 98 97 96

Library of Congress Cataloging-in-Publication Data

Umlauf, Mary Grace
    Healing Meditation / Mary Grace Umlauf.
        p.   cm. — (Nurse as healer series)
    Includes bibliographical references and index.
    ISBN 0-8273-6395-8
    1. Nursing — Psychological aspects.   2. Meditation — Therapeutic
use.   I. Title.   II. Series.
    RT86.U45   1997
    610.73'01'9 — dc20

96–14002
CIP

INTRODUCTION TO NURSE AS HEALER SERIES

LYNN KEEGAN, PhD, RN, FAAN, Series Editor

Associate Professor, School of Nursing,
University of Texas Health Science Center at San Antonio
and Director of BodyMind Systems, Temple, TX

To nurse means to care for or to nurture with compassion. Most nurses begin their formal education with this ideal. Many nurses retain this orientation after graduation, and some manage their entire careers under this guiding principle of caring. Many of us, however, tend to forget this ideal in the hectic pace of our professional and personal lives. We may become discouraged and feel a sense of burnout.

Throughout the past decade I have spoken at many conferences with thousands of nurses. Their experience of frustration and failure is quite common. These nurses feel themselves spread as pawns across a health care system too large to control or understand. In part, this may be because they have forgotten their true roles as nurse-healers.

When individuals redirect their personal vision and empower themselves, an entire pattern may begin to change. And so it is now with the nursing profession. Most of us conceptualize nursing as much more than a vocation. We are greater than our individual roles as scientists, specialists, or care deliverers. We currently search for a name to put on our new conception of the empowered nurse. The recently introduced term *nurse-healer* aptly describes the qualities of an increasing number of clinicians, educators, administrators, and nurse practitioners. Today all nurses are awakening to the realization that they have the potential for healing.

It is my feeling that most nurses, when awakened and guided to develop their own healing potential, will function both as nurses and healers. Thus, the concept of nurse as healer is born. When nurses realize they have the ability to evoke others' healing, as well as care for them, a shift of consciousness begins to occur. As individual awareness and changes in skill building occur, a collective understanding of this new concept emerges. This knowledge, along with a shift in attitudes and new kinds of behavior, allows empowered nurses to renew themselves in an expanded role. The Nurse As Healer Series is born out of the belief that nurses are ready to embrace guidance that inspires them in their journeys of empowerment. Each book in the series may stand alone or be used in complementary fashion with other books. I hope and believe that information herein will strengthen you both personally and professionally, and provide you with the help and confidence to embark upon the path of nurse-healer.

Titles in the Nurse As Healer Series:

Healing Touch: A Resource for Health Care Professionals

Healing Life's Crises: A Guide for Nurses

The Nurse's Meditative Journal

Healing Nutrition

Healing the Dying

Awareness in Healing

Creative Imagery in Nursing

Healing and the Grief Process

Healing Addictions

The Nurse as Healer

DEDICATION

This book is dedicated to the three most important people in my life—my best friend and spouse, Arthur, and my sons, Shane and Simon.

C O N T E N T S

PREFACE

This book is written for both novice and expert nurses to use as a guide for using meditation in everyday practice. To some, this topic may seem out of place with nursing. For those who have been watching the recent changes in the nature of our health care systems, the use of meditation therapy by nurses will seem perfectly logical. Although there are a number of texts on meditation for the lay reader, there is currently no such text for nurses. In addition, the interest in alternative healing methods among the lay public has also served to heighten awareness among nurses. Thus, a text written simply and expressly for nurses is very timely.

This book is part of a series of texts on holistic caring. The content is designed to meet the needs of experienced nurses who work at the bedside and also less experienced nursing students. The focus of the text is the use of the mind as a healing agent in the form of meditation. The health of our patients is multidimensional in nature. It is only appropriate that we be able to employ more than technology and manual skills to heal our patients.

Because this text is written for nurses, the level of discussion provided assumes a working knowledge of anatomy and physiology as well as the principles of health promotion. As the reader will note, the directions and information on the practice of meditation are framed primarily for the reader. Unlike many of the therapies provided by nurses, healing meditation demands that the nurse have some experiential knowledge of the practice before teaching it to patients or clients. Therefore, nurses who wish to use this therapy should practice and experience the benefits before providing this particular type of care.

The vignettes described in this book are fictionalized accounts of professional and personal encounters. None of the characters, names, or events described herein represent actual patients or persons, although the clinical scenarios are based on multiple or combined patient encounters.

A C K N O W L E D G M E N T S

Many thanks to my dear friend Dr. Lynn Keegan for giving me an opportunity to write this text and to Dr. Dorothy Fishman who assisted in reviewing the manuscript.

1 | NURSE, HEAL THY PATIENTS AND HEAL THYSELF

The practice of non-doing or just being.

Kabat-Zinn, 1990

The inward focusing of attention in order to reach a relative pure experience of the self that allows an opening into transpersonal states.

Dossey, Keegan, Kolkmeier, & Guzzetta, 1989

But another word for meditation is simply awareness. Meditation is awareness.

Levine, 1979

Margaret—Life and Death in the ICU

Margaret couldn't remember the last time she had had two days off in a row, but after tonight she would have a whole week off. Margaret had only graduated last spring, but here it was New Year's Eve, and she was already carrying a full patient load on the night shift. She had always wanted to work in ICU and had courted favor with ICU staffs during her clinical rotations. Margaret was sharp and energetic, a real self-starter. She made good grades in nursing school, but school was never like a night in ICU. As Margaret described it to her mother, working nights in a major trauma center was like working on a battlefield where you take care of the wounded from both sides of the fight.

Margaret learned a lot during orientation from the other staff. In particular, she liked to work with Sharon, the night charge nurse. Sharon had worked in ICU for seven years and easily outclassed many of the residents who passed through ICU. It was obvious to Margaret that the staff physicians trusted Sharon implicitly too. She worked harder and longer in any emergency situation than anyone else on the unit. Sharon was particularly supportive of Margaret, the newest nurse on the shift. In Margaret's opinion, Sharon was the best of the best, a role model par excellence. What a good way to begin a career in ICU nursing—working with the best!

That particular payday Friday started off innocently enough with two fresh motor vehicle accident victims being admitted by air from a big fender bender on the interstate. The night shift got the fallout of a losing battle between a little sedan and tractor-trailer. The car's passenger never had a chance, but Margaret, Sharon, and the ICU crew gave it their best for over an hour. The driver of the sedan was in better shape. He was stabilized on the unit long enough to give the orthopedists a chance to come back to the hospital and gear up for a major reconstruction. The paperwork from the patient who died had hardly settled in the out tray when another call came from the ER at about 2200 hours. They were sending in two more patients right away to bypass a logjam of semiacutes who were taking up all the ER space. The ER gave no other information except that the patients would be coming straight in with the EMT crew. No one had a chance to wonder why there was such a rush that night.

They came through the door on two gurneys covered in blood. Margaret was momentarily frozen in place as the first gurney swerved left across her path and the other went to the right into the two nearest vacant ICU bays. Along with the gurneys came a gaggle of blue uniforms and badges that swarmed and hovered over each bloody cart. The room that had been calm seconds before was filled with the shouting of vital signs, barking of orders, and the rhythmic counting of compressions. It took a few seconds to register that in that bloody mass of lines, tubes, and ambu bags were two little girls. They were maybe 11 or 12 years old and each had multiple gunshot wounds, through and through. Margaret was drawn into the throng swarming around the closest gurney and took up a position next to a sucking chest wound.

For the next hour, Margaret felt as if she were caught in a time warp. In a code, the enemy is time; some say that if you can beat the clock in the golden hour, you can cheat the devil. There were times when time seemed to stop and the bloody scene stood still. Then someone called out for the time and nearly an hour had already gushed past. During crises like these, the clock is not a useful measure of time. Sometimes the amount of bloody trash is a better gauge of progress in a code. When Margaret first tried to step back from the gurney, she was ankle deep in torn sterile wraps, shredded bloody drapes, and one continuous ribbon of EKG paper. As she picked her way backwards through the trash, she realized it was the first time she had taken her eyes off the child for the entire hour or even thought to pay attention to the parallel drama unfolding barely ten feet away.

Only ICU staff were left now. Both little girls had gone to surgery after many problems with airways and arterial bleeders. There was no more shouting and fresh crash carts were already being rolled into the unit to replace the two ransacked carts that sat gaping in the middle of the aisle. After such a long period of excitement, Margaret took a deep breath to clear her head and come back to the here and now. She felt good about this code tonight and was mentally patting herself on the back for a job well done. She looked around for Sharon, hoping for a real pat on the back from the person she admired and trusted most. There was no sign of Sharon. "Well, back to the bedside. There's no time for accolades at this hour of the morning," Margaret thought to herself.

Nearly an hour later, when it was almost dawn, Margaret finally had a chance to take "lunch." Funny, she still hadn't seen Sharon since the two little girls came through. "Maybe she got called off the unit about tonight's EMT admits," she mused. Margaret had just stepped into the break room when she noticed that the staff rest room door was closed. She sat down with her brown bag meal and tried to forget about having a full bladder. After a while it occurred to her that the door might just be closed and the rest room not occupied. She knocked twice and tried the doorknob. It was locked, but there was no answer. Margaret remembered that this door had stuck before, but she knew what to do. Without hesitation, she retrieved a letter opener from the unit clerk's desk drawer and began to jimmy the door handle.

The handle unlocked with a quick snap, but the door only swung part way open, then was stuck. In a heap on the floor was Sharon—a tourniquet was tied above her left elbow and a small trickle of blood ran down her arm.

"*A* for airway, *B* for breathing, *C* for compressions" was all Margaret could think as she dropped to her knees in the tiny space behind the bathroom door. The rest of the shift and most of the next several days merged into a blur. At Sharon's funeral, the ICU manager took Margaret aside from the rest of the staff. She instructed Margaret to report to the Employee Assistance Department at 0900 the next day. Numbly, Margaret told her manager that she wasn't sure if she was ever coming back to work. Somehow, ICU nursing just wasn't the job she had thought it would be. After all, it had killed Sharon.

Doug—Trading Places

Doug joined the Army at age 18 and served as a medic for over ten years. When he left the military, Doug went to nursing school to capitalize on the skills he had learned in the service. Although he had never seen battle, he had worked in military hospitals and in the field overseas and in the U.S. When he graduated from nursing school, he took a job at a dialysis unit and felt right at home in the semiacute environment. On the dialysis unit his leadership skills were evident and before long he was also providing backup to the transplant team. Doug liked the additional excitement of taking call and traveling at a moment's notice to retrieve donor kidneys. The additional responsibility also added to his salary, which helped at home too. By this time, Doug had two children under school age.

Like everyone on the clinic staff, Doug still took call for acute dialysis in the ICU at the trauma center. He was usually there one weekend a month. Doug wasn't particularly surprised when the senior nephrologist paged him in ICU that particular Saturday afternoon. The physicians frequently called to get a final weight and assessment on acute patients after dialysis. The mechanical-sounding voice on Doug's cell phone chirped, "Doug, the Emergency Medicine resident called. There's a potential donor for us that has just been moved to Pedi ICU, a drowning." A moment's hesitation followed. "Chances are very good that the donor is a match for our sickest dialysis patient, Mr. Ward." "What?" Doug's voice crackled back over the phone. "How can you tell at this point? I mean, how do you know so early?"

"Doug, the potential donor is Mr. Ward's only grandchild. The child doesn't have a chance; Mr. Ward does. You and Mr. Ward get along pretty well, don't you?" Another hesitation followed. "See what you can do to help the Wards through both of these events. Thanks, Doug. Call me back with the news." Suddenly, the dial tone buzzed in Doug's ear.

Doug could hardly swallow, much less say good-bye. He cleaned up his portable dialyzer and rolled it back into its miniscule storage closet. He stood there a long time, trying to make order out of the chaos of too many supplies stored in too small a space. Facing the inside of this tiny closet, he tried to create some order in his thoughts too. He thought about Mr. Ward, a good-natured, older man with polycystic kidney disease. He was a farmer, but he hadn't been on a tractor since he had started dialysis six years before. He was also a consummate grandfather. Doug had seen pictures of that only grandchild on more than one occasion. Mr. Ward's grandson was only a month older than Doug's own little boy. It occurred to Doug that there would be no more new pictures of that only grandbaby passed around during Doug's shift.

Doug had been standing in front of the open supply closet so long, one of the ICU staff jokingly asked him if he had forgotten to go home. "What? . . . no, I haven't," Doug replied vacantly as he turned the key in the lock and then headed down the hall to PICU.

Pediatric units have their own form of emotional tension when they are filled with sick children. The air is even more tense though when there is a child on life support with very little hope of recovery. There is something unreal about looking across an open pediatric unit and seeing a small child lying motionless behind the stainless steel rails of a hospital crib. Even though the ventilator's sighs and gasps create a repetitive din, it's striking when the child doesn't even flinch or rouse from all the noise. Doug tiptoed up to the crib railing and touched the child's tiny hand. All Doug could see before him was his own small son lying limply behind those steel rails.

All of a sudden, Mr. Ward was there, standing right next to Doug. Mr. Ward looked as pale as the child. Mr. Ward never even appeared to acknowledge Doug, so he hastily backed into the staff break room to emotionally regroup and decide what to do next. Finally, Doug caught the eye of one of the nursing staff passing by and pulled her into the break room with a wave of his hand. Doug blurted out, "I never thought it would come to this."

Claudia—Starting Over

Claudia thought she had left her nursing career behind when she had retired from teaching medical-surgical nursing at the local community college. Her retirement had been penciled in on her calendar for years, so it wasn't like it was a surprise. She had her testimonials and at first she wore her gold watch every day to remind her of her students. But Claudia came from the old school of nurses who were socialized to remain in perpetual motion. Although the idea of retirement sounded good, she felt more like a passive observer every day and time weighed heavily on her hands. Too many mornings she awoke at 5:45 and sat on the side of her bed wondering why she was up so early. "No clinicals and no students this morning," she would chide herself. When she was working, she used to look forward to having a day to sleep in on the weekends, but no more. Lately, she found herself looking for a reason to get up and go most days of the week. Now she told her friends that she wore her gold watch to remind herself that she did not have to go to work any more. It was much harder than she had thought it would be to slow her pace for retirement.

After one of those early awakenings, she heard the faint wail of an ambulance over the blustery sound of an early morning storm. As she peered out through her kitchen window across her still dark yard, she could see the flicker of ambulance lights on the next block. Although she barely knew those neighbors, she was immediately concerned that there was an emergency so nearby. She laughed at herself as she recalled the folktale of the retired fire horse who would run at the first sound of a fire bell. Casting folktales aside, she grabbed a sweater and slammed the kitchen door in her wake. Her brisk pace came to an abrupt halt as she stood at the open front door of her neighbor's house.

There were two EMTs in various stages of repacking supplies and a third growling into a radio as he stood on the porch. "We've

got a family member who panicked over an alarm on a malfunction-
ing IV pump for a hospice patient," he barked into the radio receiver
with some disdain. "No, we're not going to transport. We put them
on a gravity drip till hospice makes it. You know us, we're back up.
Over and out."

Just in the nick of time, Claudia remembered her neighbors'
names. Ellie, the wife, was standing at the side of a rented hospital
bed that had been erected in a living room brimming over with an
assortment of medical supplies. The husband, Bill, was much thinner
than Claudia remembered. He was lying in the rented bed attached to
a slow dripping, lone IV bag labeled "Morphine Sulphate Added."
The muted IV pump leaned forlornly against the wall and convul-
sively flashed random digital numbers alternating with the compelling
message "Get Help."

Reintroductions were in order, although the scenario was pretty
obvious to Claudia. "Hi, remember me, Claudia? I live on the other
side of your back fence. Are you both OK now?" Obviously not, but
it seemed the thing to say under the circumstances. Ellie began to cry
softly into a wrinkled handkerchief while Claudia closed the front
door behind the last EMT.

That encounter with Ellie and Bill marked the end of Claudia's
retirement and the first day of her second career. As her neighbor's
story unfolded, it was clear to Claudia that hospice was to be her
new calling. As she began to master this new role, she came to realize that, like her neighbors, her clients needed more than a store of
medical supplies and a nurse on call. Hospice care demanded different nursing skills than those she used to teach her students in medical-surgical clinicals. Now those early morning awakenings are
haunted with pondering. "If hospice has solved the dilemma of termi-
nal patients needing durable medical equipment to stay at home,
what else is missing? What kind of nontechnical care do my hospice
clients need that I can provide?"

INTRODUCTION

It is obvious that Margaret, Doug, and Claudia come fro_
ent backgrounds, have different levels of nursing experienc_ _d
work in different clinical settings. Margaret is a novice to ICU
nursing who, unfortunately, had to attempt to resuscitate a
coworker from a drug overdose. Doug is an experienced dialysis nurse who envisioned his own child in the place of a potential organ donor. Claudia knows the technical aspects of nursing
from *A* to *Z*, but knows that dying patients and their families
need more than old-fashioned "TLC" penciled in on a care plan.
Although each scenario describes different professional and personal challenges unique to the setting and the circumstances,
each of these fictitious vignettes contains a common element of
truth about the nature of nursing today.

Over the past several years, many members of our profession have developed an acute awareness of the limits of mere
technical knowledge and the limited scope of traditional nursing
therapies. Like many of us, each of the characters described in
the vignettes is more than qualified to meet the professional
expectations of their roles. However, interpersonal and intrapersonal aspects of caring demand more than technical qualifica-
tions. When faced with situations that exceed our own
intrapersonal reserves, the discomfort we experience is often persistent. Why has nursing been described as a profession that eats
its young? Being a nurse also wears on more experienced nurses
too. What are our options?

Purpose of this Book

The purpose of this book is three-fold. First and foremost, it is a
text for nurses to learn about the healing aspects of meditation
as an element of nursing practice. For many, their formal preparation as nurses did not include alternative healing methods such
as meditation. Health care has changed so much in the past five
to ten years, we are all hard pressed to keep up with many
changes in therapeutics.

Although it is not a new discovery, meditation is gaining
acceptance and is practiced more widely throughout the United

States. Nurses are now finding that they need and want information on how meditation works therapeutically. More nurses are asking questions like How does it work? What are the physical benefits to meditation? Are there risks or problems when planning to teach clients meditation? Which patients might benefit most from meditation? What is a good way to introduce this type of therapy to patients?

The second purpose of this book is to teach nurses how to meditate. Unlike many of the things nurses do to patients as part of providing care, meditation is different. We all know that the best teacher is one who has direct experience with the subject, through either intensive study or practical experience. Meditation is best taught by someone who meditates.

Nurses also have a lot of questions about the spiritual aspects of meditation. Is meditation a religious practice that is not an acceptable part of Western religions? Is meditation a sacrilegious practice? How do the mainstream religious denominations of the U.S. view meditation?

The third purpose for this text is to teach nurses how to take care of themselves. Margaret and Doug, characters described in the vignettes at the beginning of this chapter, faced this dilemma in extreme circumstances. It is no surprise that acute care nursing is challenging. Only the most skilled and knowledgeable nurses can meet that kind of demand day in and day out. Yet, how often do we overlook the emotional toll of providing care when the consequences to our actions are life and death? What are our choices when the stress becomes too much and the pain too intimate? Can we insulate ourselves from the stress and the emotional distress with apathy, or with drugs, or by simply quitting nursing altogether?

Nursing care is not simply a series of tasks or empty motions performed over the body of another human. Claudia, the former nursing instructor who is now a hospice nurse, knew enough to look past just providing physical care to her new caseload of clients. She was looking for that valuable something that only she could add to her care plans. Nursing care is provided by bio-psycho-social beings called nurses to other beings we call our clients or patients. Nurses are part and parcel of the care we provide. When our patients experience traumatic life events, we are not insulated from their experiences because we are paid caregivers. Frequently, we too are traumatized by their pain. Our daily exposure to their pain does not necessarily make us less sensitive, but it can gradually erode our intrapersonal entities. Because nursing is so physically and emotionally draining, we nurses have to be able to identify ways to rejuvenate both our bodies and our psyches to avoid burnout. Meditation is an ideal self-treatment for the stresses of nursing.

Thus, this book is written for you, the nurse, as both a potential provider and consumer of healing meditation. It is for you and for your patients.

References

Dossey, B. M., Keegan, L., Kolkmeier, L. G., & Guzzetta, C. E. (1989). *Holistic health promotion: A guide for practice* (p. 4). Rockville, MD: Aspen Publishers.

Kabat-Zinn, J. (1990). *Full catastrophe living: Using the wisdom of your body and mind to face stress, pain, and illness* (p. 8). New York: Delta.

Levine, S. (1979). *A gradual awakening* (p. 1). Garden City, NY: Anchor Books.

Chapter

2 | MEDITATION AS A NURSING THERAPY

God, grant me the serenity to accept the things I cannot change, the courage to change the things I can, and the wisdom to know the difference.

Serenity Prayer, 1951

Contemplation is the highest expression of man's intellectual and spiritual life. It is that life itself, fully awake, fully active, fully aware that it is alive.

Thomas Merton, 1961

INTRODUCTION

A great deal of what we learn as nurses and as ordinary humans we learn through experience. Sometimes the experiences are good or pleasant, although it seems that we learn the most important lessons when we are under great personal stress. Some of the strongest supporters of meditation are ordinary people who, after struggling uphill against difficult problems in life, discovered meditation. Although these people may not be particularly vocal about these struggles, occasionally they may share what they have found works for them. A few of these rare but significant occasions are illustrated in the following vignettes, which are based on real stories. You may or may not find similarities in your own life here. Do not focus on the particulars of situations described; try to look past the particular circumstances and identify what aspects of meditation may work for you or how meditation may add to your ability to meet those same types of needs among your patients or clients.

Ann—One Day at a Time

Bonnie nearly missed the driveway because the rain was coming down so hard and heavy. She had been to this AA meeting place several times before, but nothing looked the same in the driving rain. The wind and the water changed the usual landmarks, making lakes where there had been streets and rivers where there had been sidewalks. She took another deep breath to relax herself as she swung into a nearly full parking lot alongside the plain brick building.

As she created new puddles in the foyer, she was greeted by her old friend Ann, who led Bonnie to the front table. "You're on the spot tonight, aren't you Bonnie?" Ann didn't wait for an answer. "You can't tell any lies or make any excuses in this crowd," she whispered with a laugh.

Bonnie just took another deep breath and smiled. Before Bonnie could get settled in her seat, Ann had already gone back to the puddled foyer to greet more wet arrivals. Bonnie was not worried about speaking in public or about being factual. That wasn't the issue. She was concerned about truthfully portraying how her life had changed in the past five years.

As is customary, she began the meeting with, "Hi, My name is Bonnie and I'm an alcoholic." The damp crowd of smiling faces predictably replied, "Hi Bonnie." Bonnie took two more deep breaths. For an instant, she tried to tally the hundreds of meetings she had attended when she sat anonymously in the dark listening to another brave soul at the podium. She couldn't remember how many times she had thought she heard parts of her own life story spoken aloud by a complete stranger. In her five years of sobriety, she had learned how alcohol dismantles the lives of those who are addicted to it. She brought her thoughts into focus and began to tell her story without any show of emotion.

"You see me as I am today. I am 40 years old. I am single. I have a good job. I feel good and I am healthy. I have found many good friends and fellow alcoholics in AA. For all of this, I am thankful.

"Five years ago was a different story. I used to be younger. I used to be married to a really nice guy. I used to have a good job. I also used to be sick. I knew a lot of alcoholics, then too. But they were not my friends," she added quickly. "But I am thankful for all of this too. I am thankful because all my misery brought me to AA. It brought me here tonight to speak to you. For this, I am also thankful.

"We alcoholics are strange people, you know. I know you fully understand that we are addicted to alcohol and that for us alcohol became, or still is, the most important thing in our lives. We can forsake our youth. We can forsake our marriages. We can forsake our health. We can forsake our livelihoods. And we can forsake our true friends—our families—for alcohol any time of the day or night.

"There is more; let me explain it to you. When I first became sober, I thought that my life would change for the better. I bet you believe the same thing. Perhaps you have heard that AA says that they 'guarantee satisfaction.' You know, like a money-back guarantee. It's true, AA does have a guarantee. I have seen this guarantee in action. If you are not happy with the results of our 12-step program, you can have your old life back immediately." The still damp crowd jiggled with a knowing laughter.

"But when I first came into AA, I thought my life would turn around immediately. I wanted my youth back. I wanted my loving husband back. I wanted my good job back. I wanted to be healthy.

I wanted to feel good. I wanted my best friends—my family—back. All these things did not occur overnight just because I sobered up in a treatment center. I was totally distraught. At that point, I was not thankful for my sobriety. I was angry.

"The first person I really had a chance to talk to was Ann, who later became my sponsor. Poor Ann, on our first visit, I ranted and raved about how miserable it felt to be sober. Ann listened, and listened, and listened. When I had exhausted myself, I finally quit talking. Ann asked me if I was finished. I was so worn out all I could do was nod.

"Ann just sat there for about five minutes, just sat across from me and stared. Then she got up and left the room. I was totally taken off guard. I sat there like a lump. I thought she had had enough of me, had given up and left the building. Then I really started feeling sorry for myself.

"I didn't get very far down into this new pit of misery before she came back into the room almost as quickly as she had left. 'Here Bonnie, this is a special token, a coin, that we have here at AA. It's not worth money. It's actually worth more than money, but it won't buy any booze. It has the Serenity Prayer on it.' With that, she carefully placed the oversized coin in my palm and continued, 'Read the prayer when you feel the need. Give it some time, Bonnie.'

"As I read the prayer inscribed on the face of the coin, I realized that this was the first prayer I had prayed in a very, very long time. I told myself that this was a sign. I decided to take a different tactic. From then on, I always carried the coin and read the prayer when I felt like I needed to pray. Because this helped me feel better, I started to pray a lot.

"I prayed for everything. I prayed to be young again. I prayed to have my loving husband back. I prayed to be healthy. I prayed I would get a good job. I prayed to mend the rift in my family. At one point, I wrote out a list so I would not forget to pray for any of my many wants.

"But praying wasn't enough. I went back to my sponsor. I said, 'Ann, I have been praying as you instructed. I have prayed to be young again. I have prayed for my marriage. I have prayed for the perfect job. I have prayed to be healthy. I have prayed to be reunited with my family.' I showed her my prayer list in case I had left any item unmentioned.

"Ann stared at my list for the longest time and laid it on the table. Then Ann stared at me for the longest time. Suddenly, Ann got up and left the room. I was taken off guard again. This time I thought for sure she had just had enough of me, had given up, and had left the building. Then I started feeling really, really sorry for myself, worse than I had the first time.

"Again, I didn't get very far into this new cavern of misery before Ann came back into the room carrying a small pamphlet. She handed me the little booklet and said, 'Bonnie, when you pray you need to stop asking and start listening.'

"I was amazed. Do what? I thought praying was like talking, and prayers were always asking for something. Now I was staring back at Ann.

" 'Bonnie, this little book is about meditation. Read this booklet and do what it says. Meditation can be another way of praying, but it's also very healing. The difference here is that with meditation you don't talk, you just listen,' she explained very calmly.

"I had come to trust Ann's council implicitly. She seemed to understand what was going on in my head and in my heart. She was right, I was trying too hard. What I needed to do was to take things 'one day at a time.' Meditation is one way to enforce that policy each single day. Meditation has become a mainstay in my 12-step program. For this, I am also thankful.

"In closing, I am only here to tell you what has worked for me. Today, I do not worry about being young again. Today, I do not scurry after my failed marriage. Today, I do not regret that long-lost job. Today, I take care of my health. Today, I value the time I have with my family. Today, I meditate. Today, I listen more than I talk. Today, I am sober. For all of this, I am thankful. Thank all of you and thank you, Ann."

By the time Bonnie found her umbrella under the table at the front of the room, the rain had all but subsided. The lakes and rivers in the streets had receded and left the streets swept clean. As Bonnie made her way through the scattering crowd in the foyer, she heard Ann call after her as the door swung shut. She didn't catch her words before the heavy glass door closed, but she could read her lips. Bonnie thought it looked like she said, "No Bonnie, today I am thankful for you."

Gail and Joan Connect

Gail had never been much of an athlete in high school and had no time for anything else but her nursing courses in college. She had been working in ambulatory care for a couple years. Her husband Ron was a physical therapist. In general, life was good to Gail and Ron, both of whom worked the same shift at the same hospital in the rural Midwest.

Gail's work had become more stressful over the past year or so. She had recently been promoted to a managerial slot in ambulatory care, but there was talk of a merger with a regional medical center 40 miles to the north. Rumor had it that middle managers were always the losers when a big hospital merged with a smaller one. Gail unsuccessfully tried to put all the doomsaying out of her mind. When she talked to Ron about her worries, he told her that she should just do her best with the job she had.

Gail was now midway through her first pregnancy and was beginning to feel guilty about her lack of physical exercise as part of preparing for her delivery. She was very conscientious about her nutrition and was faithful in taking her prenatal vitamins every day. Still, she felt like she should have some sort of exercise plan to offset the increasing fatigue she experienced at the end of the day. Ron had always been an early morning rain-or-shine jogger and had always invited Gail to join in on his jaunts. Although Gail had made several attempts to take up jogging right after they were married, she could never keep up with her husband when he ran. She felt more like a hindrance than a companion in this activity that he enjoyed immensely. Instead, she took pleasure in having coffee ready for him when he returned at the crack of dawn each day. "Besides, the second trimester is no time to start running in the early morning darkness," she consoled herself.

Under the stress of a new round of rumors about the impending merger, Gail started having lunch with Ron in the hospital cafeteria. They were often joined at lunch by coworkers from his department. One day Ron introduced Gail to a new physical therapist on staff, Joan, who had just moved to their community. Joan and Gail immediately struck up a lively friendship. They found that they had a lot in common. In particular, Joan was a new mother. Joan had a nine-month-old daughter and was planning ahead for a second child in the near future. In an offhand way, Gail verbalized her concern about wanting to exercise but lamented that she was not mentally or physically up to jogging like Ron. There was a ready consensus among the three of them that even a routine of walking in the evening was a problem now because the weather had already begun to turn cold and windy on the plains.

"We don't have any indoor gym facilities nearby where out-of-shape pregnant nurses who work can pump iron," Gail complained in jest. "Don't worry, lifting a 20 pound toddler will build up your upper arms next year," Joan retorted playfully.

After the laughter subsided, Joan confided to Gail that she had felt the same way during her pregnancy. "I did find a way to get some physical exercise that wasn't that hard. I called it my 'no sweats' exercise. I did yoga. I took a class twice a week at the public library near where I worked. It was my way of exercising that didn't make me sweat," she laughed. Gail's interest was piqued at the notion of exercise without sweat. She leaned forward with interest as Joan continued. "And besides, I always got in my meditation time too." She paused a second as if she was mentally calculating, "Gail, I've found another yoga class nearby. I'm going to start next week. Want to go together after work?"

Gail suddenly had mixed emotions about Joan's invitation. Gail liked the idea of yoga as an exercise program, but she was taken aback when Joan mentioned meditation. "Is that your religion? I mean, are you a Buddhist or something like that?" she blurted out with some hesitation. Gail heard the ring of naiveté in her own words as soon as she said them. Almost immediately, she tried to explain her awkwardly posed query, "I've only ever lived here in the Midwest, and uh, meditation is pretty foreign. I didn't mean to pry into your religion or the way you worship. I'm sorry to be so blunt."

At first Joan didn't respond; Gail hadn't given her a chance to answer the initial question. Right on the heels of Gail's apology, Joan chuckled into her lunch napkin. "Oh, no Gail. I'm a mainstream Protestant like most of middle America. I do understand your confusion though." She caught her breath for a second, then her voice took on a lower tone. "I'll tell you the truth. I took up meditation as a way to treat the stress of my last year at college."

Joan spoke more slowly and deliberately now. "I was beginning to have panic attacks in elevators. It was happening about three times a week and it was getting worse. When I went for help at the student center, my counselor figured out that these panic attacks were brought on by a particularly stressful lab course that was on the tenth floor of the sciences building. I didn't have claustrophobia, which is what I had thought I had. Actually, I was really upset about this one course and I began to associate being in an elevator with the anxiety I felt about the course. It was the slowest elevator on campus. It felt like an endless ride up ten floors to that class that I dreaded so much.

"After a while I couldn't even use the elevator at the library or the hospital where I had clinical courses." She choked momentarily and began again. "I was really shaken by this course and these panic attacks. I thought I was going to have to quit school, until I started meditating for stress reduction. Ever since then, I meditate every day. I depend on it to keep my life in perspective. You know, some people depend on a cup of coffee to wake up. I have to have my cup of meditation," she said with a hint of a grin. "I started doing yoga when I first got pregnant and the meditation just fits in perfectly. You can do either one without the other. I'll show you how to meditate if you want to start," she said as the lilt in her voice returned.

Gail rallied with a smile, "You know, I always tell Ron that I like being a nurse because I learn something new every day. Today I learned something new at lunch. Sure, Joan, I desperately need to exercise, and I could use a little stress reduction myself. But that's another story. I'll have to tell you that one some other time. When do we start yoga?"

Joyce and Stacey—A Pact and a Plan

"You won't believe the bill I got from my pediatrician yesterday," exclaimed Stacey, the youngest of the clinic nurses sitting at the lunch table. Shaking her head, she continued, "I'm never prepared to look at the total bill. I'm just really glad that I have this job with good insurance to cover the cost of keeping my children healthy. Thank goodness it's Friday and payday." The other three nursing staff members around the table nodded in agreement with Stacey, their mouths full of lunches from home.

One by one those around the table took turns enumerating the cost of recent forays to the doctor for one thing or another. With the telling of each story, more details were elaborated and the dollar amounts multiplied.

Finally, it was Joyce's turn to commiserate with the lunch crowd. Joyce was a woman in her fifties, an LPN who had worked at the clinic longer than anyone else at the table. Joyce had oriented Stacey when she came to work at the clinic last year and had since won her friendship.

With a tone of exasperation, Joyce said, "I went to the doctor last week because I was having palpitations. I spent $1,000 in one afternoon and I don't have anything to show for it." She was pensive for a moment, then began to tap on the table to emphasize each word she said. "I had blood work. I had an echocardiogram. I had a 12-lead EKG. I had the whole works and there are probably more bills to come."

The other three only cooed with amazement until Stacey spoke up, "What did they find Joyce? Are you OK?"

"The doctor said I was having bigeminy and trigeminy, but she couldn't find any good reason for it."

Stacey pursued it further, "What are they going to do for you, Joyce?"

"Well, they've upped my antiarrhythmics one more time, which don't seem to help to begin with. And they've upped my anxiolytics, which don't seem to help me either. This doctor said that it must be anxiety. So now she wants to send me to see a specialist in anxiety disorders. Ugh, I don't like the idea of shrinks or having my head examined," she said as she began shaking her head again.

"What are your options, Joyce?" said Stacey in a therapeutic tone.

Joyce avoided Stacey's gaze and said, "I don't think I have any—except to do as I am told."

At this point, the phone began to ring in the break room, which always signaled the end of lunch. The topic of Joyce's dilemma was dropped with the first ring. Almost like robots, the staff rose from the table in unison, gathering up plastic lunch containers and half-finished drinks. All four seemed relieved that the end of the lunch hour had mercifully terminated the discussion of Joyce's problem. Each went back to her own station and resumed checking in patients or answering phones.

The lunch conversation with Joyce hung in Stacey's thoughts the rest of the afternoon. Joyce seemed so adamant about not wanting to see a psychologist. "Wasn't that even more anxiety provoking for Joyce?" she wondered. Stacey wanted to talk to Joyce in private for a minute, but the clinic was always as busy as a bus station on Friday afternoons.

The afternoon was fast and furious, as usual. It was nearly 5:00 now and Stacey had given up trying to connect with Joyce until after the weekend. She wanted to make a mental note to remember next week to get Joyce alone and follow up on today's lunch conversation. She opened her calendar to the next week and began to pencil in a note at the very bottom of Monday's schedule. It read "See Joyce/Re: anxiety."

Before she was finished writing, she heard her name being called from the far end of the corridor. It was Joyce. She waved her hand toward the back door as she said in jest, "Are you ready to go home? Let's go now or we will have to lock up tonight. Let's make the staff in Records do the honors."

"Yes, I believe it is their turn all right. One minute is all I need, Joyce. Meet you at the back door," Stacey replied.

Stacey and Joyce arrived at the back door at the same time and they pushed it closed as they left together. Joyce's car was parked right next to the back porch of the clinic and she began to unlock her door before Stacey realized it.

"Wait a second, Joyce. Do you have a minute? I was thinking about what you said at lunch. You know, about anxiety and not having options . . . ," she continued. "Has anyone talked to you about stress reduction exercises, like meditation?"

"Tests and drugs, that's all." Joyce hesitated, then said, "What do you mean meditation? Meditation for anxiety? From what I know, meditation is for hippies or gurus. Does it make you high?"

Stacey countered, "No, that's not exactly accurate. We need to talk. Meditation is just as legitimate as drugs and sometimes it works better. Like I said, we need to talk. Let's do lunch on our own Monday so we can talk. If we're busy, we'll make the time."

Joyce and Stacey made a pact for lunch and Stacey formulated a plan in her head. Monday was D-day.

MEDITATION IS . . .

In strictly behavioral terms, meditation can be described as a process developed to achieve or maintain physical and mental balance that combines the techniques of controlled breathing and focused concentration. In the words of a Buddhist monk, meditation is "mindfulness . . . taking hold of your own consciousness" (Nhat Hanh, 1975, p. 7). In the words of a modern writer, "meditation is for many a foreign concept, somehow distant and foreboding, seemingly impossible to participate in" (Levine, 1979, p. 1). Described in strictly behavioral terms, meditation seems simple enough. However, meditation is also a disciplined exercise; an exercise in strict concentration balanced with an exercise in utmost relaxation.

THE MEDITATION PROCESS

The technique of meditation couples slow deep breathing with the simple directive to mentally consider only one thought over a prescribed period of silence. The proper execution of meditation requires voluntary control to slow the rate of breathing while increasing the depth of each respiration. Again, this seems a very simple mandate. However, as a rule, we take our breathing for granted and seldom need to control it. Thus, the need to control our breathing in this way is a learned skill and takes some practice in the beginning. Once this technique is mastered, the same procedure is applied to how we deal with our consciousness.

Our thoughts are usually in constant motion. We are forever judging and entertaining any number of ideas or mental pictures in our mind's eye during every waking moment. This persistent tumbling of ideas is not necessarily a benign event to our bodies. If these ideas and mental pictures are stress producing, they trigger the stress responses of the body. As long as this barrage of ideas is incessant, the stress response is triggered constantly. Initially, the stress level may be low and the stress response relatively minor, but this activation of the alarm system may become constant. The constancy of this process becomes a habitual cycle of increasing wear and tear on the body. Therapeutically, the aim of meditation is to limit this random stream of negative stimulation and interrupt this protective mechanism gone awry.

MODERN NURSING AND ANCIENT THERAPEUTICS

Meditation is an ancient technique that can be effectively used by modern health care providers. Although state of the art medical care is known for its dependence on technology, many health problems are now being attributed to our overstressed emotional or psychic states. No amount of technology can buffer the stressors of our lives or the lives of our patients. Modern science, however, is just beginning to recognize the value of behavioral therapies in reducing the stress response. When taught to patients as a self-care skill, meditation becomes a useful and effective nursing therapy. Nurses are already responsible for the management of many symptoms, such as pain, nausea, and vomiting, that can be exacerbated by stress. Even when the patient is only expected to get partial relief from routine care, adding meditation to standard nursing practices can improve patient care outcomes.

MINDFULNESS IN MEDITATION

Although it is a special type of exercise with postures and directions, meditation is more than this. To the casual observer, meditation appears to be simply a way of resting both body and mind at the same time. However, unlike sleep, meditation does not involve shutting off consciousness to provide respite for the mind. Meditation in its truest form includes a passive attentiveness sometimes described as *mindfulness*. In the meditative state, our awareness is not allowed to ramble or be led by every sound or sight within reach. Thus, mindfulness is actually an expanded awareness that is focused, and therefore, limited.

The human environment is filled with sensory and informational stimulation. Our minds are bombarded from all directions by light, noise, vibrations, temperature, and emotions, as well as the physical sensations generated by our own bodies. Mindfulness entails learning how to take into awareness all of these forms of stimulation, without interpreting them as information. Each separate feeling or idea is simply acknowledged for what it is—sensation, noise, or intrusive thought—but it is devoid of meaning.

Many techniques are used to accomplish meditative concentration. The most well-known of these is called mindfulness of breathing. Breathing is a constant experience that carries with it no inherent emotional or intellectual connotation. As such, meditation on the act of breathing is usually recommended as one of the first meditation exercises. The beginner is instructed to fully experience each aspect of inspiration, expiration, and the pauses between each phase. In doing so, the consciousness is directed to only consider the here and now, the moment of each physical aspect of breathing.

Fully experiencing the immediate moment is also mindfulness. However, our ability to focus on the present moment is constantly challenged by our intellects. When we are children, we are rewarded for the power of our memories. As we grow older, we take in more and more information until we are in sensory overload. On top of this, we add emotional or physical challenges, such as family problems or physical illness. We quickly find that our emotional context only compounds the negative effect of the endless mental chatter inside our heads. Mindfulness is the ability to transcend the junk pile of information and our emotional overlay through focused concentration. To dwell in the immediate now, without consideration of anything outside of being mindful, is the goal of meditative practice.

Many activities can be included as exercises of mindfulness, ranging from meditating on breathing, which was mentioned previously, to the ritual tea ceremonies seen in the Orient (see chapter 5). The practice of mindfulness does not depend upon the execution of a particular set of behaviors. Any activity—walking, eating, or washing dishes—can be undertaken with mindfulness as a form of active meditation. Some cultures or religions call this mental attitude one of prayerfulness, transforming any mundane activity into an act of prayer. Mindfulness is no different in this regard. The exercise of mindfulness allows us to surpass the menial nature of the activity and connect with our higher concentrative powers through this simple activity.

ELEMENTS OF MEDITATION

Practice

In meditation, a deliberate effort is made to focus consciousness on a single idea, object, or physical sensation while being perfectly relaxed. For most people, the idea of thinking really hard while being thoroughly relaxed is an impossible task. Our culture rewards us for being active and intense. Our lives are ordered by calendars, schedules, and clocks. The concept of sitting quietly to ponder a single idea is truly shocking to our natures. This is one of the primary reasons that repeated practice is required to become accustomed to meditating. Our tendency to be overactive and overstimulated is really just a habit, and not a very good habit at that. Think of meditation as a healthy habit that becomes more beneficial with repeated use. In addition, the more stress we experience in our lives, the more we need to identify beneficial ways to reduce that stress. We know that speeding up our lives doesn't work. Alcohol doesn't work. Drugs don't work. Meditation does work, but it also requires practice.

Concentration

As most of us have observed in our own behavior, the ability to concentrate or focus our attention depends upon several factors. Children have more difficulty concentrating because they have developmental limits for attention span. As they age and practice these skills at school and at home, they begin to be able to invest more uninterrupted time in single tasks. As a rule, we facilitate concentration by providing an environment with few additional distractions. Some of us work best alone in a sparse room. Others are not too distracted by music or the presence of others nearby. Almost without exception, the ability to totally concentrate depends upon having an environment suited both to the individual and the task. The concentrative effort of meditation is no different in that regard. Meditation is best practiced in places that fit with the concentrative needs of the individual.

Environment

Privacy and a quiet atmosphere are important aspects in selecting a place to meditate regularly. In fact, using the same place and time on a daily basis is very helpful when trying to establish a meditation habit. Using the same location on a regular basis has several benefits. With continued use of the same space, the unavoidable small noises of heating and cooling systems, or dogs barking in the distance should become less noticeable. When finding a quiet place at home proves difficult, meditation music used with earphones can be very helpful to mask extraneous sounds. As might be expected, partially heard conversations of family members are particularly distracting during meditation. Fortunately, when others in the household become accustomed to the establishment of a scheduled meditation time, they will often respect this as a quiet uninterrupted time. However, the actual selection of time and place may require adjustment as inevitable distractions come and go. Again, the use of meditation music is helpful and sometimes even more effective when used with earphones to provide an additional sound barrier.

Willingness

Like any other healthy habit, meditation also demands a commitment to willingness. As with any change in lifestyle, such as beginning an exercise program, practicing that new activity must be consistent and persistent. Meditation requires the same type of regular practice as a fitness routine to improve physical strength. Muscle strength cannot be developed or maintained by following an erratic pattern of lifting weights. Physical endurance cannot be extended by an on again, off again effort to run a mile. Learning to master the powerful mental art of meditation and reap its benefits is more subtle in technique but equally demanding of willingness.

In patient education, readiness is everything. Among the thousands of people who attempt diets to lose weight, few attain their goals. Although many scientists and profiteers claim to have discovered the ultimate product, the key to success is not found in the external. The difference between successful and unsuccessful dieters is not what they eat or don't eat, or buy or don't buy. Those who succeed are completely and totally ready to make a change in their behavior.

The triggering event is probably not learning a key piece of information or buying a certain product. The underlying rationale may be obscure and difficult to put into words. The arrival at readiness sometimes reflects an individual point of saturation with feelings, not information; with a change in point of view, not a change in ability to see. Just like any other health practice, meditation is a treatment that can only be delivered by yourself. Others can control your diet by the food they prepare. If you are sick in the hospital, nurses and doctors will manage the externals of your care. But meditation is only accomplished by the willing; the reluctant are necessarily excluded from participation.

BEHAVIORAL ASPECTS OF MEDITATION

The result of active concentration combined with the control of breathing patterns produces the unique physical responses attributed to meditation. The phenomenon that occurs is in fact a behavioral treatment similar to operant conditioning or desensitization (see table 2.1). By repeated use, individuals can

Operant Conditioning	Meditation
stimulus	willingness
response	environment
	concentration
	controlled breathing
	response

TABLE 2.1   *Operant Conditioning vs. Meditation*

decondition themselves to the negative physical experience of repeated stress. It is the repeated experience of stressors that causes the body to lose its ability to extinguish the stress response. Even the most modest attempts at regular meditation deflate the body's responses to that stress. Meditation differs from operant conditioning in that individuals must necessarily deliver the treatment to themselves. The mechanism of desensitization is, however, the same as is used for the treatment of anxiety disorders. The difference in this circumstance is that the anxiety is more diffuse and the causative factors may be less well-defined.

Breathing as Behavior

One of the key aspects of why meditation yields such a positive effect on the body is related to the physical mechanisms of breathing. It is no accident that ancient peoples included controlled breathing in the technique of meditation as a healing practice. Certainly those early societies did not have the benefit of the knowledge of anatomy and physiology to understand what they observed in the human body. They learned what was effective or ineffective through repeated observation over time, the trial and error method.

The normal response of the pulmonary system to a demand for more oxygen is to increase the rate and volume of respiration while attempting to expand capacity into dead spaces. On the other hand, the intermittent and gradually progressive oxygen demands of regular physical exercise stimulate adaptive increases in circulation of the blood to the pulmonary tree. Controlled breathing that is incorporated into meditation accomplishes the same outcome. In addition, the body is simultaneously conditioned to maximize the efficiency of pulmonary circulation by slowing the heart rate to allow more time to exchange oxygen and carbon dioxide.

As we know, the body learns and can be conditioned to behave or respond to particular stimuli. Individuals who have stress-related diseases have conditions that are triggered by stress. According to our own physical makeup, we may develop high blood pressure, bleeding ulcers, heart attacks, asthma, and so on. These particular diseases are the way our bodies demonstrate what they have learned. Meditation is a method we can use to unlearn these bad behaviors using the same mechanisms that deliver the stress to our organs.

Most people believe that breathing is a totally automatic function of the body. In physiology, we learn that the brain regulates respiration according to levels of oxygen, carbon dioxide, and acidity in the blood. In a predictable fashion, increases in the rate and depth of each breath are triggered and modified by the dynamic changes in activity level and environment. In addition, we know that any type of stress can trigger an increase in both the heart and respiratory rate. As always, the brain communicates with our organs through our nervous system. Our consciousness plays a part in the process because we intellectually appraise or judge the amount of threat or stress in our daily experiences. These appraisals are communicated on a constant basis. One of the main pathways of this communication is a single nerve, the vagus nerve, which serves that excitatory purpose. In addition to one-way communication from the brain to our organs and tissues, information feedback loops also serve to relate information back to the brain. In some cases, the information relayed back is that the danger has passed or the organ is too fatigued. But this informational feedback loop can be used to override the messages sent by the brain for the body to react. It is the nature of stress diseases that certain organs begin to respond out of habit even when stress is absent. Conversely, stress may seem to be ever present and/or habitually transmitted even in the absence of actual stress.

Key Point

Meditation is a method to unlearn stress responses using the same mechanisms that deliver the stress to our organs.

Concentration

Within the higher functioning of the brain there is more than one level of consciousness. Consciousness is not a unidimensional element of brain activity. One explanation is that consciousness consists of several different areas of functioning which are described based upon their particular operations. These operational areas may be likened to the internal parts of a computer. The part of our consciousness that initially handles information is much like a microprocessor, the working part of a computer's brain. It serves as the place where everything we experience passes through, which happens quickly and fleetingly as we perceive events and ideas. Due to the tremendous volume of information that is delivered by our senses every moment of existence, none of it is stored or processed in this area of our consciousness. In the human consciousness pieces of information or sensations that hold no value decay from awareness and are lost from realization as rapidly as they arrived.

Information of current or potential relevance is taken in and appraised differently by our short-term memory. This transient function of our consciousness serves a purpose much like the RAM (random access memory) of a computer. This area of our consciousness evaluates information and makes associations between new information and stored information from our more permanent long-term memory. Some appraisals are automatic and guaranteed, such as the sensation of extreme heat. One experience with an open flame or hot surface is usually sufficient for permanent storage of causes and avoidance behaviors.

Our short-term memory is limited, however, to being able to process or retain a limited amount of information and for a limited amount of time. The same holds true in RAM computer memory; if the power to the computer is shut off the information held in this area of transient memory is lost. If the information held in our short-term memory has sufficient value it is stored in our long-term memory just as we save computer files to the hard drive or a diskette. Unlike computer data storage, the ability to retrieve detailed information from our long-term memory depends in part on the repetition of storage. Repeated recovery of the information, repeated use, repeated combination with new information, and repeated storage yields a more reliable system of information recovery. This function is what we commonly understand as the learning process.

The practice of focused concentration utilizes our short-term memory function and our long-term memory. When the body is still, the eyes closed, and the environment quiet, the consciousness is still drawing in information. Under conditions of generalized stress or illness, stress provoking information can persist by infiltrating our awareness. By attempting to control the information placed in consciousness with meditative practices, the short-term memory is prevented from considering other information. In addition, repetition of meditation gradually builds up our ability to concentrate and relax at the same time. As a result we actively condition our consciousness to exclude intrusive and distressing thoughts.

Thoughts as Things

To better understand why focused consciousness is such an important element in healing meditation, a brief review of neurology is in order. Basically, the neurological system operates using a cell called a neuron. The neuron consists of a cell body, which contains the vital organs of the cell, and a long transmitting or receiving extension called a dendrite. Neurons communicate information, such as sensations of pain or status reports of organs, from one cell to another in a chain reaction. The actual mechanism of communication occurs between the dendrite of one cell and the cell body of another. The message is delivered by means of chemical transmitters produced by the dendrite, which are delivered to receptacles on the approximating cell body. After accomplishing their work, neurochemical transmitters are immediately recycled by the cells for future use.

Neurons communicate more than body functions; they also play a role in thought processes. Each thought contemplated by the mind, for that segment of time, exists as a measurable substance—a neurotransmitter. Admittedly, individual thoughts may consist of a large number of complicated chemical sequences that we have yet to fully understand. However, the fact is that the brain must concretize each piece of information about the body and the environment to manage the functions of the body.

When we understand the basic functioning of our neural system, it is evident that thoughts do have physical form in the brain. Although they may be fleeting during their brief action between dendrite and receptor site, they do exist (Chopra, 1989, p. 84). They are chemically measurable. Scientists have identified where these complex chemicals are produced and traced their chemical functions. Knowing this, we must question the philosophical underpinnings of health care systems that address only the body.

Neural Effects

Two important physical changes occur at the cellular level in all tissues when they are regularly exercised. With consistent use, there is both improved neurological performance and improved perfusion of the tissues. These predictable improvements are directly caused by the repetition of exercise. Even after only a short period of regular exercise, dendrites can be stimulated to grow into a more dense network, providing more potential communication pathways. As the exercises are repeated, neurochemical transmitters are produced more frequently. Neurological performance increases as a function of having more pathways and the production of a larger volume of chemical neurotransmitters. Neural performance becomes faster because the network has more pathways that are accustomed to communicating in the same manner. Researchers now attribute the initial gains in performance from exercise to the overall improvement in neurological functioning that occurs early in the process.

Along the same lines, vascular changes in the tissue occur in much the same way. When tissues have to work, they require nourishment, and glucose and oxygen are delivered through the circulatory system. The increasing demand for blood supply by working tissues stimulates the growth of collateral microcirculation. As is seen frequently after heart attacks, even damaged tissues can rejuvenate when they are properly stimulated on a regular basis. These particular effects of exercise on neurological tissue persist in the same way that muscle mass persists with constant use. The principle of *Use it or lose it* holds true for all effects of exercise. Thus, the importance of daily meditation is as important as daily exercise of joints and muscles.

Although meditation was developed long before we could describe neurological functioning, meditative concentration fits with this interpretation. The purpose of concentrating with a single focus is to decondition the mind from focusing on that which generates stress. Thoughts that drain energy, aggravate, evoke frustration, or cause emotional discomfort produce disease. The physical and mental relief afforded by focusing internally promotes healing and the relief of the sensation of stress and the presence of stress symptoms. Just as physical exercise conditions muscle groups, mental exercise refashions neural pathways. With continued disuse, old pathways atrophy, just like neglected muscles.

MEDITATION AND BEHAVIOR MODIFICATION

The best technique to reduce or eliminate a bad habit is to break the cycle and put new information into the system. As we all know, the depth and rate of breathing can be controlled to some degree on a voluntary basis. This type of control is relatively easy to practice but does require concentration. Achieving control of breathing is both a skill and a talent which can be enhanced by repeated practice, as prescribed in meditation.

Science has proven that when the breathing rate is decreased and depth is increased, the heart rate also decreases. The heart not only beats more slowly, it also beats more effectively, delivering more oxygen and nutrients to the body with less effort. This technique of voluntarily controlling respirations to reduce heart rate is scientific fact. What we also know is that this physical response, slowing of the breathing and slowing of the heart, can be evoked even in the presence of acute stressors such as real physical danger and emergencies. Further, when the technique is used, the body does not transmit messages of stress to any other organs of the body. The deliberate execution of controlled breathing effectively blocks the release of stress hormones as long as the controlled breathing is maintained. Almost anyone can learn the technique of breath control alone and can employ it in any number of circumstances.

Meditation is not meant for only occasional use. The most powerful effect of meditation is the reduction of the physical symptoms of stress, but this requires the regular exercise of meditation. If we were only exposed to stress once or twice a week for 20 minutes, then an equal commitment to meditation might be all we would need. In reality, we are exposed to stress every day, all day. The strain stress places on the body becomes evident when the effect has accumulated over a long period of time. If stress could be reduced at a moment's notice, then it would not be worthy of a minute of our concern. Regular and faithful practice of meditation is required to restore current wear and tear on the physical body while giving respite to the mind. By using meditation, we recondition both mind and body, a holistic approach to a holistic problem.

SPIRITUAL AND RELIGIOUS ASPECTS OF MEDITATION

Although this text emphasizes the behavioral aspects of meditation, some readers may be concerned about the religious implications of meditation. Anyone who is sensitive about the religious significance of using meditation in the context of health care is encouraged to seek clarification from a trusted religious advisor before proceeding. Individuals with this concern should communicate directly with their minister, priest, rabbi, or spiritual advisor. In the absence of a personal advisor, hospital chaplains are experts in the spiritual aspects of health problems and issues of faith. The ensuing discussion should include a careful exploration of the particular need for guidance in employing meditation techniques for health care. As an alternative, a search of church library holdings or a religious bookstore may also turn up suitable materials for healing meditations, such as tapes and readings, that are sanctioned by various churches or denominations according to the reader's preference.

Finding new ways to augment the effectiveness of medical treatment is an important issue to health care providers and patients alike. The type of meditation, whether religious or not, is not the central issue in this book. As described elsewhere in this book, meditation has roots in many religions. The purpose of this text is to teach nurses how and when to use meditation for patient care, not to promote one religion over another. The benefits of using meditation to enhance medical treatment are sufficient justification to encourage most nurses to carefully consider using meditation for their patients. This decision, however, is up to the individual nurse.

For those readers who are interested in the religious roots of meditative practice, please consult chapter 3 for an expanded discussion of this topic.

SUMMARY

Although it is an ancient practice, meditation is a behavioral technique that is effective in reducing the ill effects of stress on the body. Meditation combines the use of breath control with mindfulness, or focused concentration, as a self-administered stress reduction therapy. When practiced on a daily basis, meditation can produce a gradual, cumulative, and preventive effect on stress disease symptoms. It is this cumulative and preventive influence that gives meditation its most powerful outcomes.

For nurses who wish to use meditation in their nursing practice, there is one important caveat. Many patients are sensitive when nurses don't practice what they preach. Nurses are not credible when teaching dietary moderation if they are overweight. Nurses who smoke are questionable when they preach to patients about smoking cessation. Meditation is a lifestyle choice just like all health behaviors. No one flosses their teeth, exercises three times a week, or avoids high-fat foods by accident. Meditation as a health practice is no different in this regard. For those who would like to teach meditation to patients, taking a class in meditation is highly recommended along with daily practice.

References

Chopra, D. (1989). *Quantum healing: Exploring the frontiers of mind/body medicine.* New York: Bantam.

Dossey, L. (1993). *Healing words.* San Francisco: Harper.

Levine, S. (1979). *A gradual awakening.* Garden City, NY: Anchor Books.

Merton, T. (1961). *New seeds of contemplation.* New York: New Directions.

Nhat Hanh, T. (1975). *The miracle of mindfulness: A manual on meditation.* Boston: Beacon Press.

Serenity Prayer (Reinhold Niebuhr, 1951). In G. Carruth & E. Ehrlich, *The Harper book of American notations.* (1988). New York: Harper & Row Publishers.

Suggested Reading

Benson, H. (1975). *The relaxation response.* New York: Avon.

Dossey, B. M., Keegan, L., Kolkmeier, L. G., & Guzzetta, C. E. (1989). *Holistic health promotion: A guide for practice.* Rockville, MD: Aspen Publishers.

Kabat-Zinn, J. (1990). *Full catastrophe living: Using the wisdom of your body and mind to face stress, pain, and illness.* New York: Delta.

LeShan, L. (1974). *How to meditate: A guide to self-discovery.* New York: Bantam.

Oyle, I. (1979). *The new American medicine show.* Santa Cruz, CA: Unity Press.

Snyder, M. (1985). *Independent nursing interventions.* New York: John Wiley & Sons.

Chapter

3

PRACTICAL QUESTIONS AND ANSWERS ABOUT MEDITATION, NURSING, AND HEALTH CARE

There have been moments in your life when you were pure awareness . . . These moments bring a sense of rightness, of total perfection, of being at-one-ment, of clarity, of feeling intimately involved with everything around you, of being free of the tension self-conscious thought brings . . . such moments are the essence of meditation.

Dass, 1978

INTRODUCTION

Simply learning a new skill does not ensure success in implementing or using that new skill. As with any form of expertise, knowing just when and how to employ a given therapy is not enough. In keeping with the goal of this book to provide a broad presentation of how meditation may be used by nurses in many settings, the following vignettes are examples of how two different nurses blended meditation into their practices. Although the bulk of the chapter provides a brief glimpse at the historical and cultural roots of meditation, it is just as important for the reader to be able to understand how these principles can be provided in the context of caregiving today. Although meditation is an ancient art of healing and spiritual practice, it is also a living art and can be an effective healing art.

Jerry—The Past and the Future in Perspective

It was in the early fall that Celia, the nurse practitioner for pediatric cardiology, met Jerry for the first time the evening after his diagnostic heart catheterization. This lanky 16 year old had been born with pulmonary atresia and had had a substantive repair at age 8. Jerry had come in for a regular checkup to get a clearance to go mountaineering with his scout troop the next summer. The routine clinic echocardiogram showed more marked changes in his heart profile. Often the normal consequence of adolescent growth causes calcification of the replacement vessel used for repairing Jerry's condition. The results of the catheterization were now final. Jerry was going to need open-heart surgery to reduce pressure in the right heart. The word from the head of the services was that the surgery should be scheduled sooner rather than later. It was standard operating procedure for the nursing staff to request a consult by Celia because patients like Jerry frequently require special handling.

As might be expected, Jerry was openly discouraged by having to undergo invasive testing when all he really wanted was to go hiking in the mountains with the rest of his troop. In the eight years since the initial repair, Jerry had been transformed mentally and physically by this newfound strength and stamina. He was no longer perpetually cyanotic and he had no recollection of how he had been limited by this condition. What he was able to vividly relate was his experience as a small child being stuck repeatedly for lab tests, the numerous failed attempts at starting IVs, the nightmarish specter of anesthesia, the panic-inducing smells of alcohol swabs and black rubber anesthesia masks, and the helplessness of being restrained and intubated in ICU after surgery.

Celia was no stranger to working with adolescents like Jerry. During the heart catheterization she had located his parents in the waiting area and was forewarned what to expect. That afternoon, Celia found Jerry still a little groggy, but obviously unhappy about the news. Her usual approach with adolescents was to introduce herself to the patient, sit down at the bedside, and explore the concerns of the patient and the parents. Depending on the results of this initial visit with the teen, she often made second visits at breakfast the next morning just before discharge. Jerry seemed too sleepy to be very engaged in the discussion so soon after the procedure. Instead, Celia gave Jerry her business card and promised to visit again in the morning.

When Celia arrived the next morning, she found Jerry's mother, who had stayed the night, just as she was leaving Jerry's room to eat breakfast in the cafeteria.

"Go ahead in. He's eaten his breakfast and is already dressed to go. I'll let the two of you talk. There's only so much a mother can do. Teenagers are so skeptical of their parents, you know. Good luck." She half-smiled and turned down the hall to the elevator.

Celia knocked twice and entered, reintroducing herself to Jerry. With a TV game show blaring, she found Jerry trying to stuff a pair of large athletic shoes into an already full overnight bag. "I'm the nurse who gave you the business card yesterday afternoon. . . . Looks like I'll be seeing you again soon, Jerry," Celia said, trying to engage him in conversation.

Jerry only nodded in reply but said nothing. The emcee on the game show continued to ply contestants with questions.

"How did things go for you yesterday? Is your leg hurting at all?" Celia pressed again and waited. Still there was no discernible response from Jerry as he repeatedly tried to force one shoe, then another unsuccessfully into the small zippered bag. Commercials for soap and deodorant provided the musical background for this test of mind over matter.

Celia stepped up to the bedside table where Jerry struggled with his improbable task. "Jerry, how about if we go down the hall and get another bag? A bag just for your shoes," Celia offered with muffled enthusiasm.

Jerry finally spoke up in a voice that was almost inaudible over the unrelenting drone of the telecast above their heads. "Do you have something that doesn't look like I've been to the hospital?" he said.

"I'm sure I do," Celia said, holding back her relief that they could escape the endless prattle coming from the television. In quick fashion, she swung open the door and ushered him into the hall. Jerry walked with a slight limp, obviously favoring the catheterization site in his right groin. Hardly a dozen steps down the hall was Celia's office, which adjoined the nurses' station on the unit. Celia unlocked her door and offered Jerry one of the stuffed chairs that sat in front of her cluttered desk.

"Sorry about the mess, Jerry. We just won't look at the desk, will we?" she offered lightheartedly. "I believe I have one of the nice shopping bags from the university bookstore down the street that should do the trick," she said as she began digging in the file drawer closest to the floor.

Celia started when she fully heard Jerry's deep voice without the sound of television to drown it out. "Am I going to have another scar on my chest? I already have one in the front and two in the back," Jerry's voice intoned ominously. She momentarily stopped her search to look him in the eye before she replied. "No, you won't." She paused again. "Is that a concern for you, Jerry?" Having just laid hands on the perfect container for the oversized athletic shoes, she handed the plastic bag to Jerry. In the same motion, she pushed the office door shut and took a seat in the other stuffed chair.

Jerry and Celia talked for more than an hour that morning. Jerry had a lot of questions and feelings about his prior surgeries and openly wondered what would happen in this next surgery. Most adolescents who have long medical histories like Jerry don't really know a lot of facts about their condition. These teens frequently have to be reeducated about what has preceded and what to expect in current treatment.

Because Jerry's memories of prior surgeries were particularly distressing, Celia decided to try something with Jerry that she had recently learned in a seminar on stress reduction. Celia was almost thinking out loud when she said, "Jerry, I would like you to try something that can help you get ready for surgery. It is something that you can use when you come back to the hospital again for your surgery."

Celia taught Jerry some simple meditation techniques and made a simple agreement with him. Jerry was going to have surgery scheduled within the next few weeks so she loaned him the meditation tape she had gotten at a stress reduction seminar to use in the interim. In turn, Jerry agreed to call Celia every Friday to report his progress. As Celia's part of the agreement, she promised to check on him before surgery and to play the meditation tape for him when he was in ICU after surgery.

Jennifer—Meditation in the First Aid Kit

This was the first time Jennifer had been able to attend a high school football game in several years. This was a special occasion because Jennifer had come to see her daughter play in the school marching band for the very first time. This was the band's first performance on the field, so excitement was high that night.

The weather had been very cool the day before, but the last vestiges of Indian summer were blowing across the freshly mowed field that night. The band marched into the stadium in full form at a brisk pace. Sequins sparkled, and the flash of dozens of polished brass instruments dazzled the attentive crowd of parents. The drummers' cadence stopped abruptly when the last of the band stood at stiff attention in their proper places in the grandstand. As a whole, they were an impressive sight in full dress uniform, white gloves, and plumed high-brimmed hats.

Jennifer also had a job to do tonight. As a rule, parents took turns helping with band performances. They moved the largest instruments on and off the marching field, and helped with uniforms and water breaks. Jennifer, a nurse by profession, was conveniently designated *the nurse* for the band that night. This meant that she was the keeper of the first aid kit, which contained basic, but necessary, supplies like tape, band-aids, and aspirin.

The evening seemed to be magically transformed by the band's fanciful costumes and the harmony of brass horns. It was so enjoyable that Jennifer almost forgot about her volunteer responsibilities until she had her first "patient." She was relieved that it was only a complaint of a headache by one of the students who had the misfortune to sit too close to the drum line. Jennifer thought to herself, "This is a great volunteer job. I can handle this."

It was nearly halftime when the band had to begin filing down onto the field to warm up. From the stands, the band students looked like a hive of worker bees. One of the band parents down on the field caught Jennifer's eye and waved to her to come down to the lower edge of the grandstand near the end zone. In the end zone, Jennifer could see a likely patient dragging her instrument across the grass. As the young woman approached, Jennifer could already hear her wheezing and coughing. She was accompanied by two other students who explained that Lisa was asthmatic, that Lisa did not have an inhaler with her, and that her parents were at home, not at the game.

Jennifer was quick to dismiss the crowd of students that was beginning to gather around Lisa. The teenagers were quick to suggest all manner of remedies and even quicker to commiserate with Lisa. Several students wanted to describe in detail their own most memorable medical emergencies, including how they had to be admitted to ICU for resuscitation or the like. Jennifer knew that the only available treatment was an ice-cold wet towel and that only one person should be occupying Lisa's attention. The crowd of sympathetic onlookers dissipated quickly when Jennifer maneuvered Lisa over to an open seat at the edge of the bleachers.

"Lisa, I'm a nurse and I've had asthma for years too. We're going to sit right here and just slow down your breathing," Jennifer said in Lisa's ear. "I know you have had these kind of attacks before and I'm sure you know what to expect. What I want you to do is to slow down your breathing."

Lisa nodded and wheezed. Jennifer got her uniform jacket off and draped the cold, wet towel around her neck. Within minutes, Lisa was pink and breathing easily. Jennifer thought, "That was easy enough. Still not a bad job."

"I just got too hot out there wearing this heavy uniform. Let me have my jacket. I can't miss this first performance," Lisa asserted as she looked around for her trumpet.

Jennifer only protested gently because Lisa recovered so quickly. Then she helped her redress to get back to the sidelines. Just like that, her patient was gone, back into the mass of blue-frocked coats and white pants.

Jennifer returned to her seat to enjoy the performance. The ten-minute routine of jazz, pop, and military tunes was lively accompaniment to the intricate patterns of marching. She could hardly recognize her own daughter in the surging lines of horns and drums. Every time she picked her out of the crowd, the line of students would weave and bob. Then she would be lost again amid the plumed hats and flashing brass. Everyone stood to applaud at the finale while the last of the students filed from the field.

Once again that same anonymous parent on the field was waving at Jennifer from the edge of the field. This time he was pointing to the 50-yard-line dugout at the center of the sidelines. Jennifer put the first aid case under her arm and picked her way through the crowd again.

On the dugout bench she found Lisa, her eyes wide with panic. Jennifer went into action just as she had before, waving off the concerned bystanders, getting Lisa's jacket off, placing the ice-cold towel around Lisa's neck, and restarting the slow deep breathing. Lisa was as white as a sheet this time though and her wheezing was much more pronounced.

"OK, Lisa, let's get this under control once and for all. Let's start where we left off," Jennifer commanded gently.

Lisa still looked panicked but nodded in agreement as Jennifer began the process again. "Lisa, you need to slow down your breathing. I want you to do what I do when I want to slow down my breathing. I want you to close your eyes. Listen to my voice and nothing else. Now, I want you to breathe along with me. Listen to me breathe in and out. Now, together let's breathe in. Slowly, . . . slowly . . . "

FITTING MEDITATION INTO YOUR PRACTICE

Although the goal of this book is to convey the practical aspects of meditation as a healing activity, it is also important to convey suitable contexts for meditative practices to be used. Nurses who choose to expand the scope of their practice with this technique should also be informed about the historical and cultural implications this choice entails. As described in the preceding vignettes, there is nothing unusual about using meditative practices in these ways.

Depending on how you incorporate meditation into your daily nursing practices, you may be asked by peers, patients, and other health professionals why you are teaching meditation. They may convey their skepticism about the appropriateness of using Eastern practices on your patients in mid-America. They may question the appropriateness of using meditation with patients who are Christians, Jews, or atheists. You may be questioned about the appropriateness of a nurse providing meditation as part of nursing care. This chapter explores the rationale behind all of these valid and likely questions that may be asked of the nurses who choose to provide meditation for their patients.

Thus, this chapter provides a brief overview of nursing within the larger contexts of healing and modern health care. For some, this discussion will only be a review of what is well-understood. For the skeptical reader, it is hoped that the discussion clarifies why meditation is well-suited to nursing practice today.

MEDITATION AND THE MODERN HEALTH CARE SYSTEM

During the present century, health care has developed from a tradition of personal service and individualized care into an impersonal corporate system built on profit and loss. This process has created economic dynasties built on technology, bureaucracy, and outmoded social roles. Today, our society is on the verge of an important change in the conceptualization of health care. Curiously, this change may both clarify and confound the practice of nursing as we know it. As the influence of technology has increased in health care, nurses have been restricted from providing low-technology care that is both therapeutic and cost-effective. High technology, not high touch, has been marketed by conventional medicine as the premier element in health care delivery.

To the dismay of the public, all technology does not cure, while much of it contributes to the misery of the disease experience. Modern medicine has evolved from the basic sciences, but it is based on symptom recognition, diagnosis, and symptom suppression. According to Nightingale (1859, p. 74), "It is often thought that medicine is the curative process. It is no such thing; medicine is the surgery of functions, as surgery proper is that of limbs and organs."

Where allopathic traditions consistently fail is in the domain of disease prevention. In addition, treatments frequently cause distress, as is evident in the vignette about Jerry presented at the beginning of this chapter. To compound this problem, the most prevalent diseases of contemporary society are those attributed to lifestyle not infectious organisms.

The modern healing sciences have evolved primarily during the current century. Prior to that time, the treatment of disease was widely practiced by laypersons, but it was often poorly understood. Nonspecific treatments were frequently provided and the sick recovered in spite of having had these often harmful remedies. Treatments of the past include the use of unrefined chemical compounds, the application of heat or poultices, blood letting, and surgical procedures, including amputations and cesarean sections. Healers and the healed may have been very pleased with the effectiveness of the potion, process, or surgery. In retrospect, however, the condition may have only been temporary in nature and due to resolve even if left unattended. Some conditions persisted even when all sorts of treatments were provided. Although our diagnostic skills are greatly enhanced with the use of x-ray, laboratory tests, and scientific skill, there are still many conditions, such as autoimmune conditions and cancer, which defy cure or control. What is evident to modern practitioners is that prevention is often the key to dealing with these types of conditions. Further, when cure is not possible, therapeutic efforts should focus on reducing the progress of the condition and preventing the inevitable suffering that accompanies most illness.

MEDITATION AS NURSING THERAPY

The specialty disciplines of nursing and medicine evolved out of the same traditional role of local folk healers. In the nineteenth century, these two healing specialties differentiated in parallel to the prevailing gender roles of the period. Nursing care behaviors were seen as consistent with the social roles of European and Western women at the turn of the nineteenth century. Medical practice was undertaken as the domain of men. The prevailing social expectations attributed to men and women carried over to the practice of nursing and medicine.

Traditional medical practice holds that the body is a cellular machine. As such, the discipline of medicine has focused on curing dysfunctions of the body; fixing that which is broken. The tenant of this paradigm, or way of thinking, is that the observable and measurable components of existence are governed by physical laws and principles. In this conceptual framework, medicine is considered a parallel science to chemistry or biology, but it is concerned with the domain of human disease processes.

To the confusion of many, nursing historically patterned itself after allopathic medicine. Only in the recent past has nursing begun to recognize its distinct professional role. Nursing has a different philosophical focus; that of caring. Nurses attend to the physical, emotional, and psychosocial needs of individuals with health challenges, as opposed to attending only to disease processes. The nursing profession employs techniques or therapies that are meant to accomplish very different goals from the medical profession.

Nursing considers the whole person, not just the diseased portion of the body. Nurses assess the developmental needs of patients and assist patients in meeting their needs. They also play a major role in the management of pain and the comfort of the dying. In addition, nurses acknowledge the health needs of the community as well as the individual or family as a unit. Nursing characteristically takes a nurturant view of individuals, constantly seeking methods to maximize abilities and enable self-care. The element of *caring*, the fundamental role of the nurse, balances the physical and emotional demands of illness or disability.

Foremost, nurses are themselves healing agents by their presence and as role models, a commodity virtually inseparable from the care provided. This phenomenon is part of the essence of nursing. The provision of nursing care is by its nature an interpersonal event. It is not the sterile and routinized process delivered as high-tech health care.

Key Point

Traditional medical practice holds that the body is a cellular machine. Nursing considers the whole person, not just the diseased portion of the body.

Nursing, Meditation, and Health Care Delivery

The use of independent nursing therapies such as meditation is consistent with the definition of nursing and the complex nature of health. The nurse is an advocate for self-care and an active agent in maintaining or improving health status. When a nurse instructs a patient in meditation, several important things happen. First, the nurse delivers a clear message regarding control. The overt intent of the nurse is to reinforce the patient's perception of control over her own health or recovery. Meditation is especially suited to this end. This therapy does not require any special equipment, and the patient can use it any time without the assistance of others. In addition, the severity of a patient's condition is not necessarily a limitation to the use of this therapy. Second, by instructing the patient in meditation, the nurse directly affirms to the patient that he is more than a physical body or a mere victim of microbes, cancerous cells, accidents, and/or congenital errors. The nurse formally recognizes and validates the patient's capability to take emotional control even when physical control may not be possible.

A New Perspective on Healing

In spite of the scientific strides made by medicine through technology, our society has begun to reexamine what the roles of technology and profitmaking in health care have done to the healing arts. As a result, many nurses (and physicians) are thoughtfully considering the therapeutic value of alternate and ancient methods of healing. Nurses are also beginning to examine their repertoire of effective and noninvasive healing skills. Nurses have always known that there is more to healing than just the use of drugs or surgery. Nursing care is necessarily a psychosocial event because it occurs as an interaction between humans. However, the social climate has been such that physicians have been the gatekeepers of service and economic reward. Thus, the modern health care system has been constructed so that payment for health care services and illness care has been assigned primarily to institutions and physicians, and for more medical technology. In doing so, our culture has discouraged the provision of preventive care and the utilization of techniques that require no technology and are low in cost.

MEDITATION AS A HEALING TECHNIQUE

Ancient healers recognized the power of the mind, or spirit. Their practices employed many therapies, including meditation, to cure, relieve, or release illnesses. From a historical perspective, we find that even archaic healing practices in different cultures share some similarities with modern medicine. In general, the art of healing consists of a system of therapies that accomplish restorative actions.

Although ancient practitioners lacked scientific knowledge, they knew that some conditions warranted treatments other than drugs, surgery, or special diets. They often employed treatments that mobilized the inner strengths of the patient. These practices have many names such as prayer, progressive relaxation, deep breathing, and meditation. These treatments are similar in method and outcome. All of them produce deep relaxation and calm the mind. Healing techniques such as meditation are commonplace in many Eastern cultures and religions. Within these cultures, the practices have served as both a preventive and ongoing treatment against stress diseases, those caused by uncertainty, conflict, and lack of control.

Healing Therapies from Eastern Traditions

The Eastern view of disease and illness incorporates a particular concept not included in the complex scheme of naming and identifying diseases used in allopathic medicine. These cultures have identified conditions not solely associated with organs or organisms but that demonstrate a lack of harmony, or balance. The importance of harmony between elements of nature and humans, and the physical and spiritual self is clearly visible in their literature and art, as well as their healing sciences.

One of their commonly used therapies, acupuncture, targets a system of pathways, or meridians, that flow through the body. Not surprisingly, these energy meridians follow a strikingly similar path to the nervous system described in physiology textbooks. Their physicians refer to this map of the energy pathways to locate where to provide the acupuncture treatments. The treatments stimulate or block the transmission of neural information from the higher centers to the extremities or organs. Modern science marveled not long ago that acupuncture provided sufficient local anesthesia for major surgical procedures with no pain or side effects. The balance of energy or feedback information within the body is viewed in Eastern cultures as a critical element to the relief of symptoms and for health in general. Meditation originates from these same cultures. Although it may be new to us, it has a longer history than we can imagine.

When the use and effectiveness of healing practices from cultures so different from our own are explained, the consumer may not be fully informed. The average person may lack the vocabulary and experience to completely understand the rationale or the mechanisms involved. In this instance, we are placed in a position to treat ourselves with a method that may not make complete sense based on our limited understanding. On the other hand, how is this different from taking a new drug or trying an experimental medical procedure? Drugs can be deadly and medications are sometimes withdrawn from the market when new harmful side effects are discovered. Surgery has many inherent risks and is simply unsuited to the treatment of stress-related illnesses and autoimmune conditions. In contrast, the potential for drug interaction or a procedural misadventure developing as a result of meditation is nil. Nor will meditation leave a permanent mark, like surgery. Meditation requires no drugs, no diets, no equipment, no expenditures, no insurance coverage, and no referrals to other providers.

ASSESSING PATIENT PROBLEMS

Although nursing employs a different perspective of health care from medicine, these two disciplines share a common concern about the etiology of illness. It is not the origin of specific diseases that is of concern; it is the mechanism that causes sickness in some people and not others. It is the perplexing appearance and disappearance of symptoms that defy treatment or cure that captures our common interest. For example, the LPN with arrhythmias in the vignette in chapter 2 presented puzzling symptoms. Although she had a complete and thorough cardiac evaluation, the root of her cardiac problem did not appear to be her heart. Her physician was astute enough to recognize that treating the heart alone would not resolve the problem.

There was a time when science had no knowledge of the existence of germs or microbes. With the invention of the microscope, scientists identified many virulent organisms attributed to contagious diseases. As science became more sophisticated, we found that the mere presence of, or exposure to, germs did not automatically cause illness. Susceptibility, in terms of immune status, was initially identified as a key factor in the development of many conditions. However, the immune system fluctuates, thereby influencing disease susceptibility. Health practitioners are just now beginning to explore the role of stress as a negative influence on immune functioning. Researchers have clarified the effect of stress on the manifestation of conditions such as hypertension and ulcers mediated by the adrenergic nervous system. However, stress is also linked to autoimmune conditions such as arthritis and lupus.

In spite of the advances of science, the stress of daily life in the twentieth century is taking its toll on our bodies. Members of our society experience the stress of multiple written and unwritten social expectations. Earning a living while dealing with a polluted and often crowded environment compounds stressor upon stressor. As a result, we must master the increasing complexity found in everyday existence. The time available for self-renewal is limited as individuals struggle for simple peace of mind in daily existence. Facing the challenge of a physical or mental illness only adds to the standard set of stressors found inside and outside our homes on a daily basis.

How Stress Affects the Body

Hans Selye (1976) described the effects of stress in his work on the General Adaptation Syndrome (GAS) or the Stress Syndrome. Today, we recognize the General Adaptation Syndrome as a factor in the development of many disease conditions. Most important are the definitions of stress and stressors that resulted from the work of Selye. Simply defined, a stressor is the causative agent or condition that exerts a demand on the organism. Stress is the resulting condition.

A stressor can be any number of circumstances, such as a need for increased vigilance, the presence of danger, or a physical challenge in any form. Further, stressors may be psychological, such as the perception of uncertainty, conflict, lack of control, or lack of information for decision making. These demands, or stressors, can be caused by extreme environmental conditions such as natural disasters or war. However, some

stressors are normal life events, such as dealing with difficult people in the workplace, raising children, or starting a new job.

Relieving Stress

Modern medicine has no drug or surgery that can eliminate stressors in the workplace or the stressors of daily life. The physical
effects of stress that accumulate over time can, however, be
reduced by counteracting the body's own protective mechanisms
that are triggered by stress. The slow deep breathing and focused
concentration of meditation help to retrain the body's functions.
By breaking the negative conditioning of repeated exposure to
stress with meditation, the body can return to its prestress state.

As a self-administered therapy, meditation can also contribute a sense of psychological control, which is often missing
from the traditional healing process. Unfortunately, patients are
too often passive participants in their own treatment. Regular
meditation, simply as a coping technique, can reduce stressor
intensity as would any active therapeutic action on the part of the
patient. Meditation is a self-care skill just like other self-care skills.
The benefits of skill building are compounded with each new
ability. With mastery of each skill, the likelihood of retaining the
current repertoire of skills is improved along with the likelihood
of successfully adding new self-care capacities.

Key Point

As a self-administered therapy, meditation can also contribute a
sense of psychological control, which is often missing from the
traditional healing process.

MEDITATION AND RELIGIOUS BELIEFS

Many patients have strong religious convictions and incorporate
spiritual practices into their daily lives. However, this important
intrapersonal resource is seldom tapped by nurses for its healing
potential. Presumably, this has been due to negative portrayals of
meditation suggesting mystical possession. In addition, many
Americans shun practices that are not commonly found within

their own ethnic customs. On top of this, the popular media usually portray meditation as an unusual practice adopted by fringe groups and only consistently found in Oriental religions.

On the contrary, Keating asserted that meditation, or *contemplative prayer*, was commonly used by Christians in Europe up until the fifteenth century (1994, p. 19). After that time, political and social forces within the Catholic church discouraged private meditation for more structured and public prayer activities. Keating asserted that contemplative prayer and meditation have seen a resurgence in the past few decades, and he is an active proponent of this practice. Keating's published works (1994) are particularly insightful and include detailed descriptions of incorporating prayer and meditative practice. Following is a brief excerpt to illustrate how meditation is operationalized from a contemporary Christian perspective:

> We begin our prayer by disposing our body. Let it be relaxed and calm, but inwardly alert . . . The root of prayer is interior silence . . . We are totally present now, with the whole of our being, in complete openness, in deep prayer. The past and future—time itself—are forgotten . . . We wait patiently; in silence, openness, and quiet attentiveness; motionless within and without. We surrender to the attraction to be still, to be loved, just to be. (pp. 136–137)

Many modern Catholics are also familiar with the works of the late Father Thomas Merton on the topic of meditation. Although he used the term *recollection* to describe the meditative process, his writings are strikingly similar to descriptions from other centuries, other countries, and other religions. Following is a small sample of his work:

> Recollection, then, makes me present to whatever is significantly real at each moment of my existence. The depths of my soul should always be recollected in God. (Merton in Mott, 1984, p. 222)
>   Recollection is a change of spiritual focus and attuning of our whole soul to what is beyond and above ourselves . . . And because spiritual things are simple, recollection is also at the same time a simplification of our state of mind and of our spiritual activity . . . True recollection is known

by its effects: peace, interior silence, tranquility of heart. The spirit that is recollected is quiet and detached, at least in its depths. (Merton in Mott, 1984, p. 217)

Over the past few decades, many Americans have become familiar with meditation through Zen Buddhism. Although Buddhism is a formal religion, the meditative practices of Zen are among the most frequently taught form of meditation taught in the United States. One of the most popular modern writers and visible proponents of Zen meditation has been Thich Nhat Hanh, a poet and Zen master. His work has the same eloquence and clear definition as that of Merton and Keating, although the religious orientation is supposed to be very different. Note the similarities of this passage by Nhat Hanh to those by Merton and Keating:

Sitting in mindfulness, both our bodies and minds can be at peace and totally relaxed. But this state of peace and relaxation differs fundamentally from the lazy, semi-conscious state of mind that one gets while resting and dozing . . . In mindfulness one is not only restful and happy, but alert and awake. Meditation is not evasion; it is a serene encounter with reality . . . Be like a lion, going forward with slow, gentle, and firm steps. Only with this kind of vigilance can you realize total awakening. (Nhat Hanh, 1975, pp. 60–61)

Although the term *meditation* is not generally found in the religious vocabulary of Judaism, many of the practices are evident. According to Donin (1972, p. 160), there is a tradition of prayer among Jews called a *service of the heart*. This tradition of daily informal and unstructured prayer has always been a consistent expectation and predates formal forms of worship. Although Judaism includes many prescribed worship services, the participants are directed to actively participate in each service. The Jewish tradition recognizes the importance of concentration to assist in attaining a sense of spiritual depth when engaging in prayer. "To assure meaningfulness in prayer, the Sages insisted upon conditions conducive to concentration (kavanah). They called for purity of thought and sanctity of place" (p. 161). Thus, there are a number of rules to follow during public services to assure a peaceful and contemplative environment.

In addition, there are many Judaic prayer practices that share characteristics of meditative practice. For example, a central element of every Jewish worship service is the Amidah, also called the Shmoneh Esrai. This series of benedictions is to be repeated morning, noon, and night. Part of the tradition of this prayer are directions on the proper execution that bear a striking resemblance to meditative methods described by others.

Admittedly, much of what we know about meditation is derived from religious contexts. However, this fact should not preclude nurses from using meditation in modern health care settings. The benefits of meditation for stress management are well-documented. Although our patients may have no control over the type and amount of stress they experience, they do possess the ability to reduce the effect of this stress on their bodies. For patients who may feel that their lives or diseases are out of control, taking control of one small aspect of their lives can become a major accomplishment. Remember, meditation is one of the few treatments that patients can use at will and that does not have to be provided by others.

Key Point

The behavioral and physical principles of meditative practice can be used by nurses to mobilize untapped inner strengths of patients without crossing religious boundaries.

REVISITING CLINICAL VIGNETTES—JERRY

The vignette describing the health challenge faced by Jerry clearly demonstrates the differences between medicine and nursing. Jerry was receiving the best medical care possible. He had the benefit of the most recent technology to precisely define the extent of his vascular problem. He had an experienced cardiologist and a top-notch surgeon scheduled to do his surgery. Celia, on the other hand, served a different role in preparing Jerry for surgery. Nurses are uniquely prepared to address the needs of the whole patient, not just the afflicted part.

Would it matter if the nurse practitioner had intervened or not? In this case, it is very likely that the combination of Jerry's developmental stage and previous experiences with surgery would have created problems with compliance in the hospital and in the home. Adolescents with chronic conditions may view not cooperating as one of the few outlets for self-determination. Educational efforts backed by reason and solid facts mean nothing to adolescents who desperately want to be like everyone else. Certainly, the expert pediatric nurse is aware of this developmental imperative. Celia made a strategic decision to offer Jerry this particular form of self-therapy. She made a judgment call based on her expert evaluation of Jerry's emotional needs and psychological readiness to participate in his own care.

Further, this vignette clearly illustrates the interactive nature of nursing care. Our patients do not experience their illnesses or health challenges in a vacuum. Many factors influence their ability and propensity to recover or master their condition. Nurses draw information from the environment and add themselves to the equation. Celia added herself to Jerry's plan of care. She became a qualitative aspect of his treatment as opposed to simply providing another quantitative treatment.

REVISITING CLINICAL VIGNETTES— JENNIFER

Jennifer's patient Lisa experienced an asthma attack while performing with a high school band during a sporting event. Fortunately, Jennifer was confident and capable in conveying the breathing techniques used in meditation to quell Lisa's symptoms. Contrary to the uninformed view of many professional and lay persons, meditation is not just a method of expanding consciousness. The fundamental elements of meditation, controlled breathing and focused concentration, create specific physical reactions in the human body. Regular practice of these methods in tandem reinforces this positive and predictable response by the body.

As a therapeutic skill, meditative techniques are an important adjunct to regular medical care. When other treatments are not available, meditation can be an important element in the nurse's repertoire. As described in this vignette, asthma attacks can occur at any time. When there is no medication available, the nurse must innovate by using the resources at hand. Jennifer used what resources she had, in this case, skills that she used herself.

As a self-care technique, meditation can serve as an important resource for patients too. Certainly, Lisa was a willing and cooperative patient under the circumstances. But it is also likely that she would be highly motivated to learn meditation as a backup to having and using her medications, *if she were taught these skills*. As a rule, nurses have to be vigilant for those teachable moments. In nursing, the teachable moment is when the patient's level of discomfort and need for new information are so perfectly balanced as to ensure adoption of what is learned.

SUMMARY

Humans are not just physical beings. The mental and emotional stressors of modern life are frequently manifested as disease conditions. The treatment of chronic and acute disease conditions also creates new forms of stress that simply complicate treatment further. Meditation is an ancient behavioral technique used to interrupt the cycle of stressor and stress response. Meditation is an effective, noninvasive therapy consistent with the nature and discipline of nursing. Meditation is well-suited as a nursing therapy because it reinforces the notion of patient self-determination in maintaining health, which is one of the foundations of nursing as a profession.

References

Dass, R. (1978). *Journey of awakening: A meditator's guidebook* (p. 4). New York: Bantam.

Donin, H. H. (1972). *To be a Jew: A guide to Jewish observance in contemporary life.* New York: Basic Books.

Keating, T. (1994). *Open mind, open heart: The contemplative dimension of the gospel.* New York: Continuum.

Mott, M. (1984). *The seven mountains of Thomas Merton.* Boston: Houghton Mifflin.

Nhat Hanh, T. (1975). *The miracle of mindfulness: A manual on meditation.* Boston: Beacon Press.

Nightingale, F. (1859). *Notes on nursing* (reprinted). Philadelphia: Edward Stern & Company.

Selye, H. (1976). *The stress of life*. New York: McGraw Hill Book Co.

Suggested Reading

Armstrong, K. (1993). *A history of God: The 4000-year quest for Judaism, Christianity and Islam*. New York: Knopf.

Oyle, I. (1979). *The new American medicine show*. Santa Cruz, CA: Unity Press.

Pelletier, K. (1977). *Mind as healer, mind as slayer*. New York: Dell Publishing.

4

INTEGRATING MEDITATION INTO NURSING PRACTICE

. . . medicine, as far as we know, assists nature to remove the obstruction, but does nothing more. And what nursing had to do in either case, is to put the patient in the best condition for nature to act upon him.

Florence Nightingale, 1859

INTRODUCTION

Although many practicing nurses have had no formal preparation on how to use meditation in their daily practices, that trend is changing. Many nursing students are personally familiar with meditation before attending nursing school, or may currently be studying alternative healing practices while in nursing school. New nurses and nurses-to-be are always concerned about how to present themselves and the skills they have to offer to their patients. In preparation for actual clinical experience, case studies are frequently used as teaching tools in nursing education. Case studies are good teaching tools because they not only present the problems faced by the patient in detail, but also describe the nurse's decision-making process and the nursing theories used to address them.

This chapter has been designed with the new nurse in mind and uses a type of case study format. Meditation is first presented in the general context of a selected number of nursing theorists.

Then each case study is described in a SOAP note format followed by a discussion of the theoretical dynamics at work in each case. Thus, the actions and decisions of nurses in different patient settings are explained in light of a suitable theoretical context. The objective of this format is not to confuse readers who are unfamiliar with nursing theory, but to clarify the clinical decision-making process for using meditation. Further, it is hoped that these case studies will better describe the who, when, where, and why of using meditation in nursing practice, rather than simply focusing on the how or what aspects. When we focus only on what to do, or how to do it, then we are truly task-oriented and ascribing to the lowest form of nursing. The best nurse is the one who knows not only the mechanics of nursing but also the art and theory of nursing.

COMBINING NURSING PRACTICE AND MEDITATION

Learning a new skill requires careful study and diligent practice. The same is true for learning how and when to use meditation in the everyday practice of nursing. The most skilled practitioners are those that are alert to developing and ongoing problems of patients. Meditation, like ·many other forms of therapy, is not meant to be used in every case or with every patient. The hallmark of an expert nurse is being able to identify the combination of circumstance and patient characteristics that lend themselves to this type of therapy. To best identify this important combination of factors, case studies are provided in this chapter. As a further introduction to clinical decision making, it is also important to discuss how meditation therapy fits with nursing theory. Many nurses are unsure of how theory fits into daily practice, thus the integration of the two is particularly important for many readers.

THE FIT BETWEEN NURSING THEORY AND MEDITATION

The discussion of meditation as a healing therapy would be incomplete without also describing how it fits within the context of nursing theory. The daily practice of nursing requires, by its very nature, the use of theoretical principles. Nursing theories provide a structure for analyzing the bio-psycho-social problems experienced by our clients or patients. These frameworks facilitate our caregiving by conceptually organizing critical information, improving collection of pertinent data, focusing information gathering efforts, and directing our decision making (see figure 4.1). Nurses add to their effectiveness by having a working knowledge of a variety of theories and conceptual frameworks. All patient care situations are not alike. Patients and their problems are unique; thus, the efficacy of nursing practice often depends upon the nurse's ability to apply abstract theoretical principles to the real-life situation. By developing a good grasp of a number of nursing theories and their potential applications, nurses are better prepared to respond to the unique needs of the client.

Much of the care provided by nurses in acute care settings is procedural and mechanistic in nature. Sterile technique, universal precautions, and the maintenance of IVs, chest tubes, and the like demand rigorous attention to the details of precisely how and when to act. These elements of acute care have their foundations in germ theory, fluid dynamics, and the gaseous exchange of oxygen and carbon dioxide. As one of the health sciences, nursing students receive intensive training in these scientific principles as they are applied to the human body. However, these theories of physical science do not constitute the science of nursing. Nursing is not solely fixed on the care of the physical body, but on the whole person, the entire family, or the

---

PATIENT PROBLEMS
Biological, Psychological, Social

NURSING THEORY

ORGANIZES	GUIDES
Thinking	Caregiving
Data Gathering	Selection of therapies
Decision Making	

FIGURE 4.1   Functions of nursing theory.

community at large. There is a separate body of knowledge that describes and directs what it is that nurses do *independently* in the provision of health care.

Key Point

Theory-based nursing care differentiates the professional practice of nursing from the menial delivery of nonspecific care.

Martha Rogers: The Science of Unitary Human Beings

In 1970, Martha Rogers began to describe and develop a conceptual model of nursing and nursing practice which was based on a new world view. Changes in world view, or *paradigm shifts*, occur when our knowledge of the universe is altered by a new understanding. The work of Martha Rogers is nursing's leading edge into that new paradigm and therefore tends to be poorly understood by many. Martha Rogers believed that the discipline of science was subject to evolution, just like living organisms. She further asserted that her work was part of that evolution (Rogers, 1986, pp. 3–8).

Until the time of her death in 1994, Rogers continued to expand and refine the elements of this model (see table 4.1). On its surface, this model appears to be less pragmatic than other theories, especially when the nurse is contextually tied to acute care practice and traditional (institutional) care settings. Many students and teachers of nursing theory balk at the apparent complexity and high level of abstraction demanded by the model. This text will not attempt to elaborate at length on Rogers' work because her work is so rich. The seriously interested reader is advised to read Rogers' own words to best capture the complexity and specificity of the theory.

It is noteworthy that Rogers' theory is very compatible with the work of Albert Einstein (Bentov, 1977; Stromberg, 1966), a mathematician, and Stephen Hawking (Hawking, 1988), a physicist. The new physics described by these scientists also speaks to the nature of matter as consisting of multiple energy fields. Notably, these energy patterns share many common principles on both the microcosmic and cosmic levels. Matter may be defined

---

Concepts

Energy fields—Both human beings and their environments are distinct, yet mutual and confluent. Energy is the true nature of human beings. Human beings are irreducible wholes that include the energy context of their environment.

Openness—The nature of the universe includes its capacity to continually be influenced by the elements within it.

Pattern—Different energy fields, both human and environmental, are distinguished by their characteristic energy signature or pattern. The nature of the pattern changes dynamically, but each human field pattern is unique.

Four-dimensionality—The universe is a nonlinear domain without attributes of space or time.

TABLE 4.1   *Martha Rogers: The Science of Unitary Human Beings*

---

by its weight or shape or other physical properties, but these are only sensory measures. At the microscopic level, matter consists of combinations of chemical elements. These elements consist of atoms which are made up of different combinations of neutrons and electrons. At the subatomic level, these animated particles are actually measures of energy. Rogers' theory does not include a discussion of the physics of energy, but it describes the nature of humans and their environments as interactive energy fields. When this elemental view of the world is appreciated, the interconnectedness of living and nonliving things becomes more apparent. This world view is indeed a striking difference from the science of cause and effect or germ theory.

In this same vein, Rogers' theory fits well with the therapy of meditation. Although the origins of meditation are very ancient, it is striking that meditation is directed at the human consciousness. Even with our advanced technologies and our sophisticated research methods, human consciousness is not well understood today. Rogers' theory maintains that humans are actually beings of energy, not just animated physical objects. Using Rogers' perspective, we can see how consciousness, human existence, the environment, and the universe are all inexorably linked. Human energy fields are confluent with and imbedded in the energy of the environment. The boundaries of these energy fields are not circumscribed; therefore, they are not mutually exclusive either.

Therefore, controlling consciousness through meditation should enable us to modify or focus our personal energy. The function of meditation is to get in touch with the energy center located in the consciousness, while the main action is to empty the consciousness of all superfluous and random thoughts. This action is both energy conserving and calming to the body and the consciousness. Through meditation, we should also be able to modify other energy fields, such as our body or our environment.

Margaret Newman: Health as Expanding Consciousness

The work of Margaret Newman (1986) is an interpretive extension of Rogers' theory regarding the concept of health. Through her own life experiences, Newman was able to operationalize health, not as the absence of a disease process, but as a higher level of consciousness. This higher level is reached in an evolutionary process of learning experiences, some of which may include physical challenges we usually call disease. These learning experiences present opportunities for the development of insight by the individual, family, or community.

Like Rogers, Newman did not acknowledge illness or disease as a central element in her theory. Both asserted that health and illness are not dichotomous conditions, one the opposite of the other. Health was described by Newman as the "underlying pattern of the person-environment" (p. 13). The recognition of patterns of behavior in context is characteristic of Newman's paradigm of health.

Newman's main focus was consciousness and its development, or expansion, throughout the life process. She asserted that health and illness are not concrete or mutually exclusive conditions or events. Under this theory, if individuals can psychically accommodate for the changes in their physical conditions, they are healthy. She negated the power of physical illness as a defining factor in health. The practice of meditation is similar in this regard. The ability to meditate and derive benefit from this practice is not limited by physical disabilities. Further, the presence of an active disease process of the body is separate and distinct from the processes of consciousness. In fact, meditation provides a means of exercising and expanding consciousness. As nurses well know, many people will not seek to change poor health

---

Basic Concepts

Unitary nature of humans and environment—Humans are centers of energy that are also confluent with the environment.

Patterning—Relatedness characterized by movement, diversity, and rhythm which is intimately involved in energy exchange and transformation. The fundamental units of analysis are space, time, and movement. The identification of patterns often requires the perspective of distance from the phenomena under scrutiny.

Health—The synthesis of disease/nondisease. Health and illness are expressions of the life process. The meaning of these phenomena is derived from an understanding of the life process as a whole.

TABLE 4.2   Margaret Newman: Health as Expanding Consciousness

habits or add beneficial behaviors until they face debilitating physical conditions. It is also possible that many individuals do not expand in consciousness until they face health challenges. It seems that health challenges may actually be a mechanism that prompts individuals to refocus from the outward to the inner. This metamorphosis of the human consciousness is the hallmark of Newman's work (see table 4.2).

Dorothea Orem: Self-Care Model

The ability to perform self-care activities is one of the central elements of nursing assessments. Functional abilities include bathing, feeding, mobilizing, and the like. All of these basic functions are required to maintain the integrity of the physical human organism. However, self-care agency also includes a cognitive component (see table 4.3). Mastery of self-care skills also indicates achievement of developmental milestones. Loss of any or all self-care skills, therefore, generates a significant emotional stressor. The resulting negative emotional effect on the individual can actually be more problematic than the loss of the particular self-care skill. As functional ability declines, the preservation of remaining skills may be seriously jeopardized by the emotional drain on stamina and effort. The motivation to challenge or prevent further functional losses becomes a critical issue in providing care (Orem, 1980).

Health-Deviation Self-Care Requisites

Seeking appropriate medical care in the event of exposure to physical or biological agents or environmental conditions associated with pathological states.

Being aware of and attending to pathological conditions and states.

Effectively carrying out therapeutic and rehabilitative measures directed to prevention, regulation, correction, or compensation for disabilities.

Modifying the self-concept in accepting oneself as being in a particular state of health and in need of care.

Learning to live with pathology in a lifestyle which promotes continued personal development.

──

TABLE 4.3   *Dorothea Orem: Self-Care Model*

From Orem, D. (1980). *Nursing: Concepts of practice* (2nd ed.). New York: McGraw-Hill.

Under Orem's model, meditation can be used as a therapy to bolster the patient's perception of self-care ability. When properly taught and presented, it becomes a therapy that patients can do for themselves. Given the nature of meditation, patients are not dependent upon any other care provider for this service. Meditation can be undertaken any time and any place regardless of the number and quality of caregiving resources available. It is immediately accessible and is not diminished by the severity of disease or the number of disabilities. Through the regular practice of meditation, cognitively intact patients will always retain this particular self-care ability.

──

WHO MAY BENEFIT FROM MEDITATION?

The decision to use meditation with a particular patient or client follows the same decision-making pathway used for other modes of treatment. All nursing actions are guided by an assessment of the patient's particular problem and, in this case, the ability to participate in the therapeutic activity. Meditation, because it requires some cognitive ability to manipulate attentiveness, is not suitable for every client. However, it is acknowledged that the professional nurse does not use every technique in her repertoire of skills on every patient in every situation. In this same vein, because each patient is unique, neither is every patient or patient problem suited to meditation.

Some nursing diagnoses are a good fit with meditation to achieve beneficial outcomes. Conditions that display a large component of anxiety, pain, or fatigue are well-suited to meditation practices to reduce the negative effects of these stressors. In addition, patient and caregiver circumstances that involve uncertainty, vigilance, or repeated health challenges are also amenable to meditative practices. Examples of these conditions are when patients are newly diagnosed, or when families are attempting to manage a condition with a predictable decline in functional ability or comfort level. Although the major action of meditation interrupts the cycle of stress hormone production that affects the body, it also provides some psychological relief from the mental stress. In some cases, the decision to offer meditation may be for the benefit of the family member(s).

Case Studies

The following case studies explore types of settings and describe patients or clients suitable for meditation as a nursing therapy. Each scenario includes a discussion of the application of nursing theory.

CASE STUDY | *The School Nurse*

Mark Applebaum is a 15-year-old middle school student who had an accident three months ago while rock climbing. He fell about thirty feet off a cliff and now has partial paraplegia of his lower extremities. He was transferred from his home school to a different school campus because he is wheelchair dependent for the time being. Mark is beginning to regain some mobility of his legs, and can resume attendance at school in a wheel-chair as healing progresses. Mark is determined to resume his former athletic activities and was instrumental in his return to school activities at this time. Mark has been back at school for one week and using the wheelchair in the crowded hallways is becoming increasingly difficult. However, he was adamant about refusing assistance from other students from the first day. Mark was discovered in the far corner of the library this morning by the librarian midway through a class period when he should have been in class elsewhere. He told the librarian that he had hurt his hand and she brought him to the school nurse to examine his injury.

Abbreviated Physical Assessment

Vital Signs—Pulse: 74; B/P: 110/80; Respirations: 20; Height: estimated at 5'4"; Weight: estimated at 100 lbs; Extremities: upper body thin and undeveloped; Affect: pleasant and cooperative but evasive in answering questions about how the injury occurred; Communication: The patient reports that he hit the knuckles of his right hand at change of classes and went to library to get out of the traffic. He also volunteered that he missed his friends from his home school, especially his best friend, and that the students at this school called him Mr. Wheels. He said that at first he was amused by the name, but after one week the name had become an ugly taunt. He also reported that he had a headache and neck ache by the end of school yesterday and could not finish all of his homework for today as a result.

Examination of Ⓡ hand: There are blue discolorations over the knuckle of the second and third fingers of his Ⓡ hand, the same findings are noted also on the

Ⓛ hand. Hands are equal in size with no swelling, crepitus, or deformity. Mild discomfort noted upon movement of either hand. Examination of head and neck: limited range of motion of head from Ⓡ to Ⓛ with report of general stiffness and pain radiating to Ⓡ shoulder. Muscles of upper arms are painful on palpation.

Problem List

- Impaired mobility—due to paraplegia
- Environment—multiple barriers to safe use of wheelchair
- Physical condition—physical demands exceed level of conditioning and muscle strength
- Social support—disruption in support system due to relocation from home school

Sample Nursing Diagnosis

- Anxiety due to impaired mobility and loss of social support.

Nursing Care Plan

- Collaborate with school counselor to modify student's class schedule to:
  1. reduce transport distances between classes
  2. allow for study hall (rest break) midday
  3. release student just before the end of class as a head start before traffic fills the halls
  4. identify peer tutor(s) for each class to assist with pacing of school work and reestablish social network.
- Consult with physical education faculty to develop a conditioning program to improve upper body strength, overall stamina, and body image.

- Conduct a nutritional assessment and diet history to identify nutritional needs to monitor hydration, maintain skin integrity, build muscle mass, and match the conditioning program.
- Schedule follow-up visits with school nurse three times a week times two weeks to monitor condition of hand(s) and build rapport.
- With parental permission, teach student meditation exercises using audiotape and tape player with music and verbal direction. Allow student to practice exercises during follow-up visits to school nurse's office.
- Explore availability of alternative type of wheelchair to accommodate for student's mobility needs and developmental status.

Theoretical Implications

Mark Applebaum is an adolescent who is facing the challenge of returning to school after being paralyzed in an accident. Developmentally, he is also making the transition from child to adult. In addition to establishing his identity as a young adult, Mark must also overcome the many social and physical barriers leading to a successful and productive life. His determination to be self-sufficient and independent is an important strength in meeting this challenge.

Margaret Newman would say that Mark has already begun to engage in an expansion of his consciousness. Although he is having some difficulty adjusting to all the changes following his accident, he still has great potential to overcome them, literally and figuratively. Fortunately, the school nurse recognized that this student was at a vulnerable juncture in his recovery. Without the nurse's intervention, Mark may have continued to flounder and struggle in a hostile predicament. According to

Dorothea Orem, with sufficient frustration, Mark might have surrendered his desire to be independent. Thus, the school nurse played a pivotal role in helping Mark begin to make initial adjustments and identify strategies to meet future demands.

Orem would say Mark's most important long-term goal is to maximize his self-care skills. Mark has to learn how to manage the physical demands of his paralysis as well as meet his developmental needs as an adolescent. Over both the short and long term, meditation can serve to destress Mark's emotional state and also help him focus his inner strength. Mark's paralysis will always demand more psychic and physical energy than usual to accommodate his loss. However, by using meditation, Mark will be able to conserve and focus his energy to achieve and maintain his highest level of wellness.

CASE STUDY | *The Oncology Nurse*

With every first visit to the outpatient oncology treatment area, the nurse manager conducts a brief intake interview with all patients. The newest patient, Ben Walker—a recently divorced 37-year-old black male postal carrier, was diagnosed with cancer of the lung approximately three years ago. Initially, he received three rounds of chemotherapy and radiation. He was apparently in remission in the interim until he developed two localized areas of acute pain (right femur and right ischial spine). He was able to work through most of his previous treatments but now complains of difficulty in ambulation. He has just completed a bone scan which suggests metastasis of the lung cancer to the bone. Ben has declined further chemotherapy and has declined participation in group therapy sessions provided for patients. He is to begin radiation therapy as a drop-in immediately and daily thereafter until a course of 21 treatments is complete. Ben arrived for treatment alone and apparently drove himself to the clinic.

Abbreviated Physical Assessment

Vital Signs: Pulse 80 and bounding; B/P: 140/90; Respirations: 26; Height: 6'2"; Weight: 205; Skin: warm, moist, hands perspiring; Extremities: slight tremor of hands; Affect: alert, cooperative, and apprehensive; Speech: noticeable tremor in voice, halting speech patterns; Mobility: moves slowly in ambulation and transferring, favoring his right leg; Communication: The patient wants to know when he can return to work and when the pain will relent. He also mentions that he wants to spend time in outdoor activities with his 10-year-old son when school lets out in three weeks. Medical History: denies HTN. Additional observation from the radiotherapist: It was necessary to tape Ben's leg to the table due to his tremor, which became more pronounced during the procedure.

Problem List

- Anxiety
- Pain from bony metastasis
- Insufficient emotional and/or social support

Sample Nursing Diagnosis

- Anxiety due to disease status and lack of social support.

Nursing Care Plan

- Review techniques being used by Ben for pain management. Verify dosage routine that will provide sufficient coverage until radiation is expected to relieve symptoms. Review potential side effects of medications and need for communication about effectiveness or problems to treatment team.

- Fully describe procedures for radiotherapy and expected outcomes of the treatment and provide written instructional materials. Reinforce this teaching and solicit questions on subsequent treatment visits. Provide direct-line phone number to clinic as backup for questions or concerns.

- Provide one-to-one instruction of meditation technique beginning immediately and continuing over next five visits.

- With the collaboration of the radiotherapists, schedule Ben's regular visits to occur as first treatment given after lunch. Allow Ben to sit in the quiet treatment area to meditate and relax before the actual treatment.

- Introduce Ben to the tape library services of the treatment center. Provide a list of suggested relaxation/meditation tapes to borrow and use.

- Collaborate with the house social worker to explore with Ben possible sources of social support for him. Discuss plans for his care should his health decline or should he become unable to work.

- Contact the volunteer arm of the local American Cancer Society to inquire about identifying a cancer survivor to match Ben's gender and ethnicity. With Ben's permission, arrange for the volunteer to meet him for coffee at the clinic cafeteria when pain reduction has been established.
- Monitor B/P every other visit for persistence of elevation as noted on the first visit. Use this opportunity to spend one-to-one time with Ben to establish/maintain rapport and continue assessment.

Theoretical Implications

Ben has been managing his health challenge well prior to this recent setback. Although his condition has taken a turn for the worse, Ben is trying to maintain control by delaying or refusing treatment that may be beneficial to him. In view of Newman's theory, Ben may be emotionally detached from himself and others. It is not apparent to the nurse if he has any personal support system during this difficult time. She has seen no evidence that he feels safe to explore his own feelings or ask for help. The nurse recognizes that Ben's condition may worsen in the near future. Without a caring network, he may succumb to his disease prematurely.

On the other hand, Ben's desire to retain control of his care is a behavior of survivors. The nurse recognizes the delicate balance between supporting self-care initiatives and offering support services. Properly presented, meditation can do both. Meditation can be marketed to the patient as a self-administered therapy to reduce his stress level and enhance the action of his pain medication. The nurse should carefully explain to Ben how meditation will allow him to conserve his physical and mental energies for the time he spends with his son and for work. If he wishes, he can ask the clinic chaplain to meditate with him during his visits over the next few weeks. In any case, meditation can be an ongoing self-care activity in spite of the severity of Ben's condition.

CASE STUDY | *The Home Health Nurse*

The Visiting Nurse Association has just received a consultation for Jose and Juanita Vega as clients. Jose is an 84-year-old retired university faculty member who was diagnosed with dementia four years ago. On his last physician's visit, he had a recorded weight loss of 23 lbs over approximately six months. At this time, he is unable to handle money, drive a car, select his clothing, or go out unaccompanied. Recently, he has been sleeping irregularly and has become reluctant to bathe in spite of Juanita's gentle persuasion. Juanita is a relatively active 82-year-old woman who had her right knee replaced two years ago. Until recently Juanita was able to take a walk daily in the neighborhood for exercise. However, as Jose's condition has deteriorated, she has needed to supervise him almost constantly. They have six grown children, the nearest of whom lives 30 miles away. As a result Juanita is virtually the sole caregiver for her husband. According to Jose's neurologist, Juanita has also apparently lost weight involuntarily during this same period due to this responsibility. Juanita's only complaint is that she can no longer attend church services, nor participate in the Women's Guild.

Abbreviated Physical Assessment of Juanita

Vital Signs: Pulse: 90 and regular; Respirations: 24; B/P: 120/100; Height: 5'7", Weight: 122; Skin: warm and dry with notable extra skin folds from upper arms; Affect: alert and very pleasant but apologizes for lack of makeup and casual clothing; Appearance: neatly dressed, but clothing apparently oversized and secured at side with safety pin; Mobility: uses cane to ambulate; Medical History: denies previous history of HTN; acknowledges weight loss but attributes this to combination of intolerance to standing for long periods to prepare food and the need to constantly monitor her husband.

Problem List for Juanita

- Weight loss
- Possible hypertension
- Stress, both physical and emotional

Sample Nursing Diagnosis

- Actual and potential stress due to caregiver responsibilities for spouse with Alzheimer's-type dementia as evidenced by weight loss and verifying statements.

Nursing Care Plan

- Visit weekly for one month.
- Monitor B/P and weight on subsequent visits (referral for B/P to follow elevations in three serial readings).
- Request diet consultation from Visiting Nurse Association (VNA) dietician.

- Refer to local Alzheimer's Association for respite visits by volunteers; request ASAP review.
- Schedule VNA home health aides on Monday, Wednesday, Friday schedule to assist with bathing and personal care of Jose to begin Monday next.
- Refer to Meals on Wheels to supplement Juanita's ability to prepare at least one main meal Monday through Friday.
- Refer to social services arm of Juanita's church for midday meal supplements in interim before intake completed by Meals on Wheels; also request pastoral visitation.
- Instruction in meditation as stress reduction technique.

Theoretical Implications

Although Jose is the patient with the medical diagnosis, the home health nurse has very little to offer him directly. Juanita, however, is her husband's main caregiver. Should something happen to her health, neither would be able to live independently in their own home. According to Rogers' theory, the energy fields of both Jose and Juanita are inexorably linked. His every need must be met by her. As his condition declines, her energy demand only increases. Without nursing interventions to bolster the environment and support Juanita, the condition of both will only spiral downward.

Although Juanita is not sick, the nurse is correct in identifying preventive actions for her in the nursing care plan. Juanita has been so focused on the care of her husband that she has all but forgotten to care for herself.

A simple way to help Juanita to remember to care for herself is to teach her to meditate daily. The nurse can explain to Juanita that along with good nutrition, she must get sufficient rest to be able to keep up with Jose's care. Given her motivation to keep her husband at home, Juanita is very likely to give meditation a try if it will help in this regard. Orem's model would support using meditation in this way to meet the needs of the patient-family member caregiving dyad. Especially among the elderly, there is a delicate balance between their physical abilities and the demands of day and night care. However, when family members are highly motivated the nurse's job is much easier. In this case, Juanita's attentiveness to her husband may be refocused to also meet her needs through meditation.

CASE STUDY | *The Nurse Practitioner*

Jeannette Robbins has a severe headache and has come to an urban neighborhood primary care clinic operated by the county health department located adjacent to a public housing project. Jeannette is a 42-year-old black female. She is single and has a 14-year-old daughter who attends school. For the past four years, she has been a full-time office worker, working 45–60 hours a week. She is employed through the XYZ Temporaries Agency, but is paid a minimum wage and receives no benefits such as overtime, sick leave, or health insurance. Jeannette's clinic record reflects that she is hypertensive and is currently taking two antihypertensives. Jeannette relates that she has been trying to find a better job. She had located another temporary job on her own that would at least eliminate her long commute by bus to her present work assignment. However, the mandatory preemployment training for the new job was scheduled for that very day, which conflicted with her current temporary assignment. She states that she wanted very much to attend the training but feared that she would lose her job with the temporary employment service. Her headache had developed the previous afternoon and was so severe by that morning that she was unable to go to work at all.

Abbreviated Physical Assessment of Jeannette

Vital Signs—Pulse: 84 and regular; Respirations: 22; B/P: 220/105; Height: 5'3"; Weight: 147; Skin: warm and dry; Affect: alert, shields eyes from light, seated in patient waiting area bent forward and holding wet cloth to forehead; Appearance: casually dressed, clean, and neat, unaccompanied to clinic; Medical History: history of migraine headaches and HTN; Pain Assessment: unilateral sensation of extreme pressure on right side of head, originates at orbit and extends posteriorly to occipital region, increases on ambulation and with exposure to bright light, intermittent nausea without vomiting when pain is intense, onset of mild symptoms in afternoon of previous day, increasing to severe (9 on a scale of 1–10) during night and early AM, unrelieved by OTC analgesics (800 mg generic Ibuprofen) with approximately 5 doses over past 20 hours.

Problem List for Jeannette

- Hypertensive crisis—urgent
- Migraine-type headache symptoms
- Stress, emotional

Sample Nursing Diagnosis

- Pain due to hypertensive crisis and/or migraine headache.

Urgent Nursing Care Plan: Immediate

- Urgent Care Hypertension Protocol for Nurse Practitioners (clinic protocol)
    1. Procardia 10 mg, gel capsule pierced with needle, placed sublingual, NOW.
    2. Monitor B/P Q 10 minutes for 30 minutes.
    3. If B/P not WNL (within normal limits) after 30 minutes, call EMS for transport to county ER.
- Migraine symptoms
    1. Place patient in quiet, darkened area.
    2. Place patient in supine position.
    3. Provide wet cloth for forehead.
    4. Monitor for resolution of headache symptoms with normalization of B/P.

Outcome of Immediate Care

After receiving Procardia sublingual, Jeannette's blood pressure came down to 140/90 and her headache pain was significantly relieved.

Nursing Care Plan: After Resolution of HTN Crisis

- Hypertension
    1. Review hypertensive medications; validate dosing schedule and drug availability with patient.
    2. Consult with collaborating physician regarding crisis and dosage.

3. Schedule for weekly B/P monitoring during Nurse Practitioner's own clinic through next month.

4. Instruct patient in stress identification and stress reduction techniques, including meditation.

Theoretical Implications

It was clear to the nurse practitioner that Jeannette's hypertensive crisis was not simply an exacerbation of her hypertension. The nurse practitioner accurately identified that Jeannette was experiencing a considerable amount of stress from a number of sources. For example, although Jeannette is a dependable worker, she is not highly skilled and earns only a minimum wage with no benefits. Economically, she lives from paycheck to paycheck and is in constant fear of being without work. This fear is so great it has hampered her ability to obtain a more permanent or more rewarding position. Jeannette stated that taking time to search for another job will cause her to be fired by the agency that gives her temporary assignments. Unfortunately, the combination of these events, the migraine symptoms, plus the hypertensive emergency, and the aborted attempt to get a better job could easily reinforce Jeannette's sense of fear and hopelessness.

It is interesting though that this combination of events may have other implications for Jeannette. After her blood pressure had normalized, Jeannette and the nurse practitioner had a few minutes together alone. In effect Jeannette said, "While lying here in the dark with this wet cloth on my head, I've been thinking. I have decided something. I am going to have to do something different. I don't know what, but this doesn't work."

This astute nurse practitioner understood what Jeannette was trying to articulate. Jeannette had just realized that her headache and elevated blood pressure were not accidental symptoms. It was becoming clear to her that she did not have an effective way to manage the stress in her life. Her stress had assumed physical dimensions and could prove to be lethal.

According to Margaret Newman's theory, Jeannette had an experience that expanded her consciousness. She had gained insight into the nature of her own condition. It had suddenly become clear to Jeannette that her body was expressing her emotional distress through her physical symptoms. Many people, nurses included, never truly believe or understand that there is a direct relationship between the mind and the body. Fortunately, Jeannette experienced this revelation in the midst of a reversible and temporary health crisis.

This knowledgeable nurse practitioner further recognized that Jeannette's revelation was evidence of readiness. Jeannette was ready to do something different, to make a change in her life, and she was ready to learn new behavior. All the well-meaning health teaching in the world is worthless if the proposed student is not ready to learn. Whatever the nurse believes is important to the health and happiness of a given patient is irrelevant. Patients operate in their own belief system and associate importance with utility. The subject of the teaching has to match the patient's understanding of events and his goals. Jeannette's revelation signaled an important window of opportunity for the nurse practitioner to teach her new coping strategies as well as techniques to control her symptoms. Based on Jeannette's own statement, the nurse practitioner would be wise to use the current clinic visit and subsequent follow-up visits to teach Jeannette meditation and other stress-reduction techniques.

CASE STUDY | *You, the Nurse*

Nurses, like you, who work directly with patients daily encounter disabilities, disease, and sometimes death. Our patient's day-to-day reality is often filled with anxiety, fear of the unknown, and physical pain. Witnessing the toll that disease takes on patients and their families also takes an emotional toll on those of us who work with them. The emotional demand is even greater when nurses are vested in the curative process, one that is intent on conquering disabilities, disease, and death. The curative process is often not sufficient to reverse the harm of many conditions. Medications may not be sufficient to relieve pain. Then, death is the great equalizer of young and old, rich and poor, the well-cared for and the neglected. We nurses often experience a personal disappointment in not being able to resolve all the problems recorded on the care plan.

Nurses are not insulated by their professional roles from identifying with the patients whom they serve. We are most deeply touched by the patients who resemble someone in our own lives, or even ourselves. It seems that as we accrue more time working with patients, it is harder to disassociate ourselves from them. It becomes easier to identify the common denominators of our existence, the simple elements of comfort, rest, working, playing, and laughing. These simple things are often out of reach of patients. This touches us in a very personal way. We nurses often feel guilty when we leave work for the day to go home. It's called the guilt of survivorship. The sick cannot walk away from their disease like we can walk away from our jobs. As nurses, we face that cruel irony more frequently than we will readily admit.

In spite of the technical preparation nurses have, it is a superficial training for empathetic caregiving. At graduation from nursing school, we end our formal preparation and begin again as students of our patients. It is with repeated exposure to patients coping with illness and death that we begin to comprehend and internalize their experiences. Repeated encounters with another's reality seasons and tempers our sterile academic preparation. As a result, our caring consciousness is fashioned and shaped by our patients. Our metamorphosis is not without a personal cost. Caring is not unidirectional. It is dynamic and demanding, inherently imbalanced, and favoring the patient.

Nursing care presents a unique set of demands to provide precise technical care as well as an empathetic personal interaction. However, to survive professionally, each nurse must identify a mechanism for renewing this inner resource. Our caring sensitivity is the hallmark of nursing. Those nurses who cannot rejuvenate their stores of personal energy often display burnout. Burnout has been described as a condition where the nurse can no longer care about patients. The emotional interaction becomes too personal and too constant to continue without respite.

Problem List for the Nurse

- Burnout—Burnout becomes obvious when nurses avoid investing time in patients. Nurses with burnout frequently display indifference to patients or their concerns or assert wide personal distances. They also habitually spend more time handling the patient's medical records or giving direction to other staff. As a result, there follows a general lack of attention to detail or to individualizing care. Errors in medication administration or failure to note important changes in patient status are likely the result of habituated indifference to patients.

Sample Nursing Diagnosis

- Potential and actual depletion of psychic caring abilities (not currently listed by the North American Nursing Diagnosis Association).

Nursing Care Plan for Self

- Develop additional skills in the nontechnical aspects of nursing: counseling, therapeutic communication, behavior modification (meditation), instructional methods, and grief therapy.
- Identify and regularly employ mechanisms such as meditation, counseling, or artistic expression to enhance personal energies, center those energies, and replenish them.

Theoretical Implications

As we nurses have gained awareness of our true nature as caregivers, the obligation we have to ourselves has become clearer. Burnout should not be viewed as the inevitable outcome of doing a good job of caring for our patients. Neither should burnout behaviors be tolerated among our peers. We should refuse to believe that the hallmark of a nursing career is that it is short-lived, like serving a term in the Peace Corps. A nursing career is not simply a process of psycho-emotional catharsis selected by those with a burning need to serve humankind. The burnout experienced by nurses is not a cathartic process signaling the end of a career. The rejuvenation of our inner selves, the recovery of what has been spent is also part of the healing process. The therapeutic presence that we nurses bring to the bedside needs to be fed and nurtured just like that of our patients.

Key Point

Nurses must be able to recoup the energies expended in providing nursing care.

SUMMARY

Theories of nursing guide the practice of nurses. Regardless of practice setting, there are a number of theories or models that are applicable to the patients or clients that nurses serve. This chapter provideds a brief overview of works from only three theorists that fit well with meditation. Meditation can be effective in reducing the physical manifestations of stress for patients. It can also be an effective tool for nurses to use to refocus their own inner energies. Caring for patients is more than giving injections and dosing pills; it is an interpersonal interaction. The constant psychic drain of providing care can deplete the nurse's ability to continue caring. The self-care benefits of meditative practice are evident for both patients and nurses. Both groups can use it to care for themselves.

References

Bentov, I. (1977). *Stalking the wild pendulum: On the mechanics of consciousness.* Rochester, VT: Destiny Books.

Hawking, S. (1988). *A brief history of time: From the big bang to black holes.* New York: Bantam Books.

Newman, M. (1986). *Health as expanding consciousness.* St. Louis: C. V. Mosby.

Nightingale, F. (1859). *Notes on nursing* (reprinted). Philadelphia: Edward Stern & Company.

Orem, D. (1980). *Nursing: Concepts of practice* (2nd ed.). New York: McGraw-Hill.

Rogers, M. (1986). In V. M. Malinski, *Explorations on Martha Rogers science of unitary human beings.* Norwalk, CT: Appleton-Century-Crofts.

Stromberg, G. (1966). *A scientist's view of man, mind and universe.* Los Angeles: Science of Mind Pub.

Suggested Reading

Dossey, B. M., Keegan, L., Guzetta, C. E., & Kolkmeier, L. G. (1988). *Holisic nursing: A handbook for practice.* Rockville, MD: Aspen Publishers.

Dossey, B. M., Keegan, L., Kolkmeier, L. G., & Guzzetta, C. E. (1989). *Holistic health promotion: A guide for practice.* Rockville, MD: Aspen Publishers.

Fawcett, J. (1985). *Analysis and evaluation of conceptual models of nursing.* Philadelphia: F. A. Davis.

Snyder, M. (1985). *Independent nursing interventions.* New York: John Wiley & Sons.

Chapter

5 | HOW TO BEGIN MEDITATING

*For nowhere, either with more quiet or more freedom
from trouble, does a man retire than into his own
soul, particularly when he has within him such
thoughts that by looking into them he is immediately
in perfect tranquility; . . . Constantly then give to
thyself this retreat, and renew thyself . . .*

Marcus Aurelius, 121–180 A.D.

INTRODUCTION

For some people, just getting started is a challenge. Meditation is one of those things that is very forgiving of mistakes the novice may encounter. Finding the proper combination of time and circumstance is not nearly as important as the willingness to begin. Thus, the following suggestions are just that, suggestions. If something works for you, then it is satisfactory. There is no right or wrong way to meditate. Read on, but don't hold back just because things aren't just right at the moment.

SELECTING THE PROPER TIME AND PLACE

When and where to meditate is most important when trying to develop the habit of meditation. Regularity of practice will also depend, to some degree, on the others in your household. Select a time and place conducive to the concentration of meditation and try to stick to it. Inform your family members that you have set aside this short period daily for your meditation. If you like, your more mature family members may join you in meditation, but only if they also plan to give serious effort to it. In the beginning, it is important to be selective about when and where you meditate to better ensure the results you desire most.

When?

The best time to meditate is when there will be fewest distractions. For people who live with other people, the hour before the household awakens is an ideal period of quiet. This suggestion is well-suited to those people who are naturally more alert and energetic in the morning. For those who are not morning people, it is better to avoid the inevitable fatigue of late evening hours. In the morning hours, the body will be rested and more likely to be able to maintain alertness even with relaxation. In addition, the ability to concentrate is usually better before the day begins because there are fewer things circulating in the consciousness.

How Much?

It is not necessary to set aside more than 15 to 20 minutes for meditation when beginning to practice meditation. Do not be overambitious and expect to be comfortable meditating for an hour at a time when you have just begun. Start with these shorter time periods and work up to longer periods as you grow with meditation.

On the other hand, 15 minutes may seem like an eternity for many beginners. Try to stick to the time you have allotted even if your concentration is poor or you are greatly distracted.

If you give up too quickly, you will defeat your own initiative to practice regularly. If you allow your family to roust you from meditation time, you may give the impression that you are not serious about this activity. Be patient and persistent with yourself. Allow yourself time to gently master this new and beneficial habit.

Where?

The best place for meditation is one that is conducive to concentration; that is, one that presents few visual distractions, or at least will allow the use of an object for visual focus. When you are just beginning to establish a regular practice meditation, it may seem difficult to identify the best combination of time and place. Do not be overly concerned about finding the perfect place. Simply make the best of your situation and move on to making meditation a habitual practice.

If necessary, be creative. For example, some people meditate in their car at home. Cars do provide some acoustical insulation and usually have good tape players. The only precaution in this technique is to avoid running the car engine in closed spaces (garages) and to avoid parking in desolate areas without locking the car doors. Otherwise, the automobile may serve as one of the most private and comfortable locations readily available to most people.

As you gain experience in meditating you will be able to meditate in spite of noises or the usual rumble of family life. In the beginning, however, look for a space that is peaceful and accessible. Later, you will be able to meditate wherever you feel comfortable, or whenever you especially need to destress. You may also want to identify a place at work to meditate during your workday. A park bench in front of a fountain can be a delightful pleasure for a 10-minute midday meditation. Most hospitals have chapels, which are well-suited to people seeking peace and quiet on a busy day.

Timing Yourself

By now you are probably wondering how to meditate for 15 minutes if you have your eyes closed and are truly meditating.

This is a good question and the answer is very simple. You use a clock. Any clock that is quiet or does not tick too loudly can be placed where you can easily see it when meditating. It should not be placed where you have to turn your head or body to see the time. When you want to know the time, you can gently open your eyes, check the time, and close your eyes again. The ability to estimate time during meditation will come with repeated practice. Keeping on a time schedule is always more of a concern to beginners than to experts. In any case, do not worry about how long you are spending in meditation. Worry about making meditation a daily practice.

COMFORTABLE POSITIONING

There is no requirement that meditation must be done while assuming a particular position. We have all seen photos of yoga masters contorted in a myriad of ways we could never imagine for our own bodies. Erase those images from your mind. Meditation does not require contortion, only absolute relaxation. For beginners, it is only important to find a position that can be maintained for the entire meditation period without having to break concentration to alleviate discomfort. Because the initial steps leading into actual meditation involve relaxation procedures, try to avoid the recumbent position during beginning sessions. As the level of relaxation increases, the novice may end up asleep before achieving the meditative state.

Sitting

It is usually best to begin meditation exercises in a sitting position. Sitting upright will allow the maximal amount of mental attention while achieving maximal physical relaxation. The upper body should be erect or supported in an almost ninety-degree angle. The common description of how to accomplish this posture is to visualize that the top of the head is attached to a string suspended from the ceiling. The taut string lifts the head, neck, and spine into alignment. The shoulders should be level with the floor to enable the chest to inflate easily with each deep breath.

However, the overall posture is meant to be relaxed and not rigid. A straight-back chair is useful to maintain this position. Alternatives to this are sitting on the floor, up against a wall with a pillow at the small of the back, or up against an upholstered couch. It is easy to maintain this straight, although relaxed, posture when breathing exercises are used consistently throughout meditation. If you find that you are bending forward or leaning to one side during meditation, use the deep breathing process to reclaim a proper posture gradually over three or four breaths. If any adjustments in posture are needed during practice, just be sure to correct your posture slowly and gently. Make all movements slow and deliberate so as to retain the physical attitude of relaxation and serenity.

Placement of Arms and Hands

The arms should be allowed to lie comfortably next to the body, or to rest gently on the upper surface of each thigh. The hands should lie palm open, in an upward position, without touching each other. The reason for using this particular hand position is because the hands and fingers can easily become a distracting source of tactile information. By their nature, the hands are just like the eyes in their ability to identify shapes and surfaces. They, too, are constantly seeking information and want to do so when we try to quiet our other senses. As we attempt to quiet our thoughts, the mind looks to its usual sources of information for distraction. Keeping the hands open and facing upward eliminates this particular source of mental amusement and communication. Keeping the palms of your hands facing upward is the equivalent of closing your eyes or turning off the lights to reduce stimulation.

Eyes—Open or Closed?

There is no particular rule of meditation that requires the eyes to be closed or open. Again, assume the position of greatest comfort and least distraction for you. If sleepiness, regardless of time of day or how you sit, is a problem, then keeping the eyes open may be necessary. However, distraction can also be reduced if the eyes are trained on an inanimate object that does not move. Some people like to focus their attention on a candle flame in a semidarkened room. This particular technique seems to soothe some people, but it may not always be feasible in institutions or settings where oxygen is used or fire regulations do not permit open flames. However, a small battery-operated flashlight pointed toward the ceiling can work just as well when a candle is not feasible.

It is worth rementioning here that using a candle in a darkened room has no particular spiritual or religious function. Darkening the room and using only one limited source of light does, however, effectively eliminate visible clutter, thereby reducing visual distraction to a minimum. Use whatever method works best for you and is most comfortable for you based on your own particular situation.

Body Position

For individuals with particular health problems, the nurse should encourage appropriate body positioning according to the usual standards of care. For example, patients with acute cardiovascular problems should be encouraged to assume a position with the feet elevated to prevent dependent edema. COPD patients will be more comfortable if they are allowed to lean forward with their arms resting on a table. All of the usual accommodations of care should be consistently provided and simply interwoven into the recommendations provided for meditative practice.

Foremost, the best position for meditation is one that works well. With repeated testing, the right balance of position, tension, and relaxation will become evident. When something doesn't work, try something else until the fit is good. Repeated practice also wears away the sensation of awkwardness that is so apparent when meditation is being learned. This is the reason there are repeated suggestions in this text to repeatedly try a number of activities as part of regular practice. It is not necessary to use only a single type of meditation, although it may not be helpful to change techniques too frequently. Variety is the spice of life, but it can also be distracting. Just keep in mind that meditative practice should be calming and soothing, not necessarily entertaining or distracting by its variety of experiences.

STARTING THE PROCESS

The following exercise is designed for beginners who have had little or no prior experience with meditation. The object of this brief exercise is simply to become accustomed to what a brief meditation feels like. Many people find sitting motionless to be an unusual experience for them. Americans are more accustomed to watching television, reading, doing needlework, or praying while sitting quietly. Meditation removes even those somewhat passive activities. Thus, you may have to get used to focusing your concentration on your body or your breathing. This may take a little getting used to, but with patience and repeated experience, it will become easier to be relaxed in your own silence.

Read through the following exercise completely before going through with it. This first meditation exercise is described in detail to clarify different behaviors and sensations. Review these directions again when you finish and then again periodically to reinforce all aspects of the technique as you continue to practice daily.

A Beginner's Exercise

The purpose of this exercise is to briefly explore meditation on your own. This exercise does not require special music or the need to have it read aloud to you. These are basic instructions on the mechanics of the process. Go slowly and do not be concerned if you have forgotten the exact sequence of events. Simply allow yourself about 10–15 minutes and enough patience to meditate or just relax for the full period. When you are finished, avoid jumping to your feet or rushing off to the next activity. Try to retain the soothing effect of each meditation activity.

When You Are Ready

- Assume your position of comfort in the place of your choice whenever you are ready to start.

- Proceed gently with each activity and without rushing. This race is not for the hare, it is for the tortoise.

- Take a slow, full deep breath without overinflating the lungs. This is called an in-breath. The lungs are filled not just from the expansion of the chest but also from the abdomen.

- During each inspiration, feel how the air moves inward through your nose, over your soft airways, through the bronchi, traveling to the lungs.

- Create a mental picture of how the air fills that space in your lungs. Watch how it swirls while it inflates even the smallest spaces.

- Hold that first breath, gently, for just a few seconds. Then release your breath slowly and evenly through your mouth. This is called an out-breath. The cycle of one in-breath and one out-breath is called one full breath or one complete breath.

- Feel the air move slowly across your air passages, across your tongue, and out your lips. Remember, in meditation, breathing is meant to be both a nourishing and sensory event.

- Feel the movement of your abdomen as your lungs fill with air and become empty again.

- Continue this process of slow breathing with total concentration. Pay close attention to how breathing feels, how the moving air feels, and the effects breathing has on your body as a whole.

- Do not be concerned about what you think you are supposed to do, or see, or feel. Just experience this natural event, over and over again.

- Experience your breathing and do not allow thoughts and ideas to distract you from concentrating on your breath. Continue monitoring your breathing, nothing else, for your full allotment of time.

- You may feel that your breathing efforts are jerky or uneven. Do not try to seize control of your breathing. Just try to slow down the mechanical steps of breathing. Practice will smooth out the rough edges over the first several weeks.

- As a beginner, you should only be concerned about investing the bulk of the effort in focusing and refocusing concentration on the breathing. After that, everything will fall into place.

- When you have meditated on your breathing for your targeted amount of time, you may discontinue the exercise by gently opening your eyes.

- Gently reawaken your body with some gentle stretching exercises before arising to your feet. Make the transition from meditation to the balance of your day a calm and peaceful process.

- Try to retain the tranquil physical and mental aftereffects of meditation practice as long as possible after each exercise session. Try smiling for a change. This is, after all, the usual objective of meditation.

Introductory Progressive Relaxation Exercise

The following meditation is provided as a structured activity for the person who is new to meditation and relaxation exercises. This particular exercise is also designed to be read aloud to others or audiotaped for personal use. Each step in the exercise is described separately in great detail. This particular exercise is meant to be used regularly at the beginning of each meditation period. This format is used because maximal benefit from meditation depends upon being able to internalize, not just recount, each step.

When you are prepared to begin, assume a comfortable position. Follow each of the instructions as directed. Do not hurry or rush through them. Please note that the following exercise contains many separate instructions (marked with bullets) and some contain pauses (written in parentheses). If this exercise is read aloud for a group meditation, the reader should allow the length of two or three complete breaths between each separate instruction. Each pause should allow enough time to elapse for one complete breath (one in-breath and one out-breath). Thus, the periods of silence between instructions are longer than the periods of silence between statements within an instruction. This will assure that the pace is sufficiently slow but even for beginners. When the exercise is complete, slow stretching exercises are recommended before resuming regular activities.

When You Are Ready

- This is a special time for you, a time of meditation, a time of peace and relaxation. Softly, easily, let your eyes gently drift closed.

- Use your breathing to center yourself. Breathe deeply in and then deeply out. (pause) Slowly in, and slowly out.

- Release the thoughts and concerns of the outside world. (pause) Let your breathing be your guide for this meditation. (pause) Slowly in and slowly out. (pause) Slowly in and slowly out.

- As you breathe in, you can feel a powerful and calming energy flow into your lungs with each breath.

- As you exhale, each out-breath takes with it all your tension and fatigue. (pause) All that is left is perfect relaxation and a feeling of great peace.

- Feel that calming energy flow in like the crest of a wave with each in-breath. (pause) As certainly and calmly as it rushes in, it flows back out again in one cleansing sweep.

- Breathing in, breathing out, (pause) feel your whole body relaxing and releasing tension with every breath, (pause) releasing worry with every breath.

- Feel the gentle sensation of your clothing upon your skin. (pause) Feel the rhythmic sensation of your breathing.

- Still gently breathing in and breathing out, bring your attention to your feet.* (pause) In your mind's eye, visualize the calming energy flowing in, flowing like waves on the shore.

- Feel that energy surging through your body to your feet and back out again, taking with it all tension and stress.*

- Breathing in and breathing out, let your attention move upward to your legs. (pause) Feel the weight of your legs.* (pause) Feel how your breathing energizes your legs while drawing out any tension or fatigue.

- The waves of energy from your in-breathing continue to rush down through your legs and feet.

- The warm yet tranquil waves wash away all tension. (pause) Each breath brings new refreshment, each wave becomes a surge of peaceful warm energy.

- It is now time to end the exercise. You may now return your concentration to your breathing. (pause) You may now slowly open your eyes.

NOTE: To progressively relax the entire body, repeat the preceding instructions marked with an asterisk (*) and insert the names of other parts of your body (arms and hands, torso and back, head and neck). Move the focus of relaxation from the feet toward the head. Depending on how long the exercise is planned to be, additional time can be used for meditating on breathing alone.

PROBLEM SOLVING

Typically, when you first begin meditating, everything feels awkward. Do not be discouraged because you feel restless or distracted. With continued practice, these irritations will gradually fade into the background. Suggestions for other difficulties are as follows.

Muscular Tension

If you sense that there is some tension in a particular area of the body such as the neck, a slow and gentle range-of-motion exercise may be necessary to release some of the tension. Range-of-motion exercises should be limited to a slow stretching effort to avoid hypermobility of a joint or muscle group already affected by injury, disease, or stress. It is also useful to take a warm bath just before attempting meditation and relaxation activities. Standing in a warm shower has a very soothing effect which can be enhanced by taking a number of deep breaths at the same time. For those who live alone, standing in a warm shower is the next best thing to having a massage. Anyone can close the bathroom door, turn on some music with a slow tempo, and get away for just a few minutes. Even when a meditation is not feasible in a busy household due to circumstances beyond your control, take a break and head for the shower.

Immobility

Immobile body parts, such as limbs affected by stroke or immobilized by traction, may respond to a gentle and superficial massage. Stroking the skin over the target area can also help to relieve muscle tension when deep massage is not indicated.

High Stress

When stress levels are high, just getting into the mode of relaxation is difficult. At these times, it may be necessary to allow extra time to get ready to fully relax. This time investment, which is essentially a cooling off period, may include a warm shower or sitting and reading for five to ten minutes. Avoid smoking or drinking caffeinated beverages immediately before meditation or relaxation activities. Both nicotine and caffeine are stimulants which will make meditating and relaxing harder to accomplish.

THE MENTAL ASPECTS OF MEDITATION

The main expenditure of mental energy should be placed upon a singular thought, idea, or mental picture of your choosing. While trying to develop a habit of meditation, it may be preferable to use the same focus for an extended period. It is the nature of the mind to act like a television which presents an unrelenting series of partially related thoughts and pictures. Avoid getting drawn into the melodrama of your chattering mind. Gently and calmly refocus your concentration as many times as is necessary during your designated meditation time (see table 5.1). Consider it your mental calisthenics to develop your mental fitness routine.

1. Passively acknowledge the intrusion by the invading thought.

2. Do not follow this thought or add to it.

3. Avoid traveling with your stream of consciousness.

4. Bring your mind's eye back to the original focus.

5. Repeat this process as many times as is necessary.

6. Take no account of how many times this occurs.

7. Consider each return to the point of focus as a mark of success.

8. Repeat these successes as many times as necessary.

TABLE 5.1   How to Refocus Concentration

Being Mindful of Your Breathing

Beginners may find it easiest to concentrate on their breathing and not focus on thoughts or ideas. On first reading, this statement may seem confusing. The period of meditation that follows the relaxation of the body is devoted to experiencing the physical act of breathing. This particular technique allows the beginner to use a sensory experience to assist in concentrating. The act of breathing is a unique tactile experience that is usually overlooked as a pleasurable activity. Although focusing on breathing is recommended for beginners, it is the traditional technique regularly used by the religious masters of the East. In this case, what works well for the novice is what also works well for the experienced teacher.

Breathing should be deliberately slowed in rate but increased in depth. There should be a longer pause in the cycle of breathing when the lungs are full than when the lungs are empty. The movement of air in and out of the lungs offers a variety of sensory experiences throughout each breath cycle. The ability to savor the sensation is much better when the rate is slow and unhurried.

As breathing is slowed and each breath deepened, the heart rate will also slow down. Contrary to first impression, there is no danger in reducing the pace of pumping. Although the lower limit for heart rate is about 60 beats per minute, cardiac effectiveness, the heart's pumping ability, actually increases as the heart rate slows. When the heart has more time to fill each contraction, it is more efficient. Better efficiency also reduces cardiac muscle fatigue. Along with improving cardiac efficiency, slower blood flow spends more time in the pulmonary circulatory system. With the greater lung expansion, improved air exchange, and reduced heart rate, there is more time for oxygen and carbon dioxide exchange to occur. The ultimate result of the introduction of controlled breathing is improved oxygen supply to the entire body.

The regular practice of focusing on breathing is an excellent introductory activity to begin focusing concentration on affected body parts. The sensation of energy and warmth that accompanies controlled breathing can be focused on stiffness or muscle tension as well as sources of pain or dysfunctional organs.

REGULAR PRACTICE

Nothing can compare with daily practice. It does not matter if the subject is typing, speaking French, or learning to ride a bicycle. Daily practice or daily exercise is the best way to ensure the best results. It is difficult, however, to acquire new habits no matter how beneficial they may be. There is no doubt that discipline is required to use meditation on a regular basis (see table 5.2). Unlike many healthful activities, the immediate feedback, such as weight loss or muscle strength, does not appear. We commonly use cues like these to reinforce new behavior and judge its effectiveness. When we do not have those types of information as feedback, it is easy to lose motivation.

Meditation is different in this regard. It is less common to see meditation used to affect external measures, such as weight or muscle strength. The effects of meditation are usually seen on a different level, from a more holistic perspective. For individuals with cardiovascular problems, they may experience a gradual decrease in pulse rate or blood pressure. For others, there may be a similar gradual reduction in anxiety level. Daily stressors may appear to be reduced in potency or effect. If meditation is focused on the reduction of pain or to improve the function of a particular part of the body, those very outcomes may occur. If

Step 1   Decide to meditate for a set period of time each day.

Step 2   Assume a comfortable position.

Step 3   Take slow, deep breaths.

Step 4   Sequentially relax each part of your body.

Step 5   Focus your concentration.

TABLE 5.2   *Developing the Meditation Habit*

the goal of meditation is to improve overall health, that may be measured by fewer colds or fewer days of illness per year. Therefore, the kind of changes that may occur as a result of regular meditation must be identified on an individual basis. These outcomes should be used as positive feedback to maintain a regular schedule of meditation.

Some people find it helpful to attend group meditation sessions held at churches or other community centers. The stimulation of doing the exercises in a group can provide additional motivation and deter feelings of boredom from practicing alone. Humans are social animals and seem to prefer doing things in groups, even if it just means sitting in a circle and not speaking.

IMPROPER TECHNIQUE

After reading this text, the average individual should be able to begin meditation on her own or to instruct others in basic techniques. Inevitably, some people are concerned about technique. What if I do it wrong? they ask. The most important aspects of meditation as a technique for self-healing are described in order of importance in table 5.3.

Group Classes

If you find that healing meditation is a particularly difficult goal to achieve alone, many community education programs offer classes on meditation. These classes are often provided by experienced persons who conduct classes in a group format. These

Breathing	Breathe deeply at a slow regular pace.
Body position	Assume the position most comfortable for you that will allow you to stay awake.
Concentration	Center your thoughts on your breathing; aids to concentration include soothing music or training your eyes on an inanimate object or a point of light in a darkened room.
Start slowly	Begin with meditation periods of only 5–10 minutes and spend about half that time going through the steps to relax each body part.

TABLE 5.3   The Basics of Meditation

classes are useful to gain additional perspectives on what works for others. In addition, some hospital chaplains may be able to provide meditation sessions in the hospital chapel if sufficient demand can be established.

Using Meditations on Audiotape

In the beginning, some people find it beneficial to use taped exercises because they provide consistency while practicing. Using an audiotape is also a dependable method to elicit the desired behavioral response each time you meditate. Any method that can be used to minimize distraction, including the variation of your own working memory of the process, is desirable. While building the habit of daily meditation, all efforts should be taken to avoid the distractions of any novelty in method. In this case, the aim is to habituate, to build a habit, for the physical and mental aspects of meditation and relaxation.

In addition, many novice meditators are concerned about how long to meditate. An audiotape will provide a consistent gauge of pace and how much time has transpired by its very length. As the meditation period lengthens, new tapes can be readily made to accommodate that change and any personal preferences in methods and techniques as you go along. Thus, home-produced tapes may actually have some advantages over commercially made products which are widely available.

Please note that no special training is needed to be able to read the exercises in this book while audiotaping. As long as the speaker's words are clear and the voice is gentle, this is sufficient. The pace of delivery should be unhurried, observing the pauses noted in the text. At minimum, a pause is the length of time required for one complete breath, which includes in-breathing and out-breathing one time each. As an additional guide to pacing the exercise the reader should also follow each element of instruction while doing the reading. It is often helpful to audiotape while reading an exercise or series of exercises while someone else is actually meditating. This provides a more natural, relaxed delivery and seems to eliminate much of the self-consciousness involved with speaking into a microphone.

SUMMARY

This chapter describes only the most basic aspects of meditative practice. It is not uncommon to feel awkward sitting in one position while trying very hard to do nothing on purpose. Most nurses are used to a busy pace and initially have difficulty sitting still. This is predictable and should not be interpreted as a major failing. On the contrary, comfort with the process and mastery of the basic mechanics of breathing and relaxation only come with practice. Thus, the instructions provided in this chapter should be reviewed several times to establish a good foundation for the exercises that follow in the next chapter. In addition, there are many good books on meditation listed in the Suggested Reading section for this chapter and at the end of this text. Readers should not limit their sources about meditation to this text alone.

For those nurses who wish to teach meditation techniques to their patients, it is preferable to use a written outline or script when teaching to avoid overlooking any important instructions. As an aid to readers, the meditations found in this chapter and the next are provided in a clip-out format (look for the scissors ✂) in the appendix. Thus, the exercises may be removed from the back of the book without destroying the text itself. Like any other type of student, patients appreciate having an outline of any materials discussed in class or copies of exercises to help them practice at home. After mastering the basics of meditation, review this chapter and adjust the content of the exercises to fit the learning needs of your particular patient population.

References

Aurelius, M. In Long, G. (1957). *Meditations of Marcus Aurelius.* Mount Vernon, NY: Peter Pauper Press.

Suggested Reading

Benson, H. (1975). *The relaxation response.* New York: Avon.

Moyers, B. (1993). *Healing and the mind.* New York: Doubleday.

Novak, J. (1989). *How to meditate.* Nevada City, CA: Crystal Clarity Publishers.

6

INTRODUCTORY GUIDED MEDITATIONS AND MEDITATION EXERCISES

Peace, be still.

Psalm, 46:10

What we are is to be sought in the invisible depths of our own being, not in our outward reflection in our own acts.

Thomas Merton, 1955

In the midst of the deepest stillness, God speaks to us His Word. And indeed, He does so in the purest and noblest place the soul has to offer, in her essence. The perfect quiet prevails: neither creature nor image ever gain access to it.

Meister Eckhart, 1979

INTRODUCTION—BASIC MEDITATION

Among the many advantages of meditation are its flexibility and simple principles. Meditation can fit into any lifestyle and can be incorporated into daily routines. Meditation does not require special clothes or special equipment. You do not have to travel to a special place at a prescribed time on a prescribed day. You do not have to memorize any special words or sayings. You do not have to be physically fit or have any special athletic or mental skills. You do not have to be initiated or pay dues either. Although there are many ways to meditate, there are very few wrong ways to meditate. Everything you need to meditate you have close at hand at all times.

Practice

In order to derive optimal benefits from meditation, it is important to practice on a regular basis. Although it is often difficult to learn new habits, meditation is not a habit that you will later need to break. When meditation is practiced on a daily basis, at the same time and in the same place, the initial awkwardness will dissipate. The time we invest in meditation becomes just another aspect of how we care for ourselves, like bathing and grooming. These peaceful interludes become a form of indulgence that rejuvenates and refreshes.

Environment

Carefully select the time and place for your regular practice of meditation. Avoid changing either when trying to develop your meditation habit. It is nice to have a special place to get away to meditate, but fancy trappings will not have any affect on your satisfaction or your progress. You may find that you appreciate having a comfortable cushion, a book of special readings such as the Bible or the Koran, and a single tape of meditation music. But these things are not particularly important in meditative practice. You already possess all that you need to begin the experience if you are willing and faithful to your practice.

Willingness

Trying something once is easy. Making a permanent change in your lifestyle is not so easy. At first, it may be hard to remember to set aside the time to meditate even when you are willing.

However, like any good health habit, it can be restarted repeatedly without harm. Meditation is not a behavior that occurs by accident. It is purposeful and planned. Plan to do your meditation immediately before or after some other good health habit. Make a conscious effort to link your practice with something as regular as, for example, your morning shower or brushing your teeth. Think about scheduling your meditation to immediately follow this event each morning. People seldom forget to shower or brush their teeth each morning. These hygiene and grooming activities are pleasant activities and that simple pleasure of feeling clean and fresh lingers for some time afterward. Meditation is well-suited to follow a simple and predictable activity like brushing your teeth. After a period of weeks, you will begin to associate the two events and seldom forget the new part of your morning self-care ritual.

Mindfulness

The elements of practice, environment, and willingness will add to your ability to become mindful in your meditation. Keep in mind, however, that mindfulness is a gentle and peaceful experience. There is nothing forceful or compelling about this aspect of meditation. For each thought or intrusive sensation that you experience, simply acknowledge it and permit it to drift aside. Even though there will be many mental and auditory intrusions into your time of contemplation, do not become discouraged or disturbed. Let persistence outweigh the number of distractions in your meditation. Focus on the experience of the moment in time you currently occupy. In this space in time, there is no other time before or afterward. Being mindful is something everyone can do if they take the time and effort.

EXERCISES AND TECHNIQUES FOR BEGINNERS

Many techniques can be used in the process of meditation. Techniques, in themselves, are not meditation. These techniques are simply methods used to focus concentration and quiet the mind. Meditation can be anything you want it to be—a time of prayer, a healing experience, or a form of fitness training. How you go about it is up to you. Consider the following exercises just as you would the many types of exercises for physical training. Riding a bicycle, swimming, and lifting weights are different types of exercises, but all have a common outcome, physical fitness. Each activity exercises different parts of the body in different ways. The following meditation exercises are not different. Try several techniques once or twice in the beginning, then select one or two techniques that seem to work for you. Use these one or two techniques exclusively for a period before adding other exercises or discarding an earlier technique. The idea is to allow yourself some variety without putting yourself on a revolving schedule. Keep your meditation periods and the exercises as simple as possible. Your meditation should be structured yet uncomplicated.

The exercises described in this chapter are to be used after you have gone through the beginning relaxation exercises described in the previous chapter. This process may take longer during periods of high stress. Do not rush yourself through the meditation process. Take as long as necessary to become totally relaxed and centered before beginning other techniques. Do not be discouraged if on some days you have great difficulty in reaching this point. Be patient with yourself and commit to a minimum amount of time for practice. In the beginning it is not uncommon for the period of initial relaxation to be longer than the period of focused contemplation or meditation. Remember, like anything special, if everyone could do it, it would not be very special.

MINDFULNESS OF BREATHING

Breathing is such a common and automatic experience that we seldom give any thought to it. From the moment of birth, breathing is part of our nature. For the most part, the rate and depth are perfectly and automatically regulated by the brain. However, we also possess the ability to voluntarily slow down and speed up the rate. In doing so, we either increase or decrease, respectively, the volume of air we are able to accommodate. From a simply mechanical point of view, the objective in this particular exercise is to slow the rate of breathing and therefore increase the volume in each breath.

For those who are new to meditation, emptying the mind may seem an impossible task. One way to counter making the mind empty is to fill the mind with that of your choosing. There are a number of ways to use the breath in meditation; some of them follow.

Technique 1: Counting the Breath

In the counting method, each breath is counted from one to ten. You may use any number of techniques to fill each period of inspiration and expiration with counting. If you find your mind wandering at any point in counting, stop and start over with the number one again.

When You Are Ready

- In your mind's eye, visualize the number one at some distance from your body.

- When you slowly inhale, visualize this number being sucked into your lungs with the air you breathe.

- Picture the number one entering your nose, passing through your upper airways, down into your lungs, and mixing with the air in your lungs.

- Watch this number being exhaled back through your airways and out through your lips. Waiting before you now for your second breath is the number two.

- Imagine that this number becomes your second breath and travels the path of your breathing.

- Give each breath its own identity. Do not allow yourself to slur the details of how each breath travels into your lungs and out again.

- Occupy your mind with the details of each aspect of each respiratory event.

- For each intrusion of wandering thoughts, recognize them and allow them to pass from your consciousness.

- Return your concentration to your breathing whenever you are ready to finish and thus complete the meditation.

NOTE: Whenever your counting concentration is broken, gently return to number one and start over again. Do not be discouraged regardless of the number of times you must start over without being able to reach number ten. It is a true discipline for even experienced meditators to count successfully to ten.

Technique 2: Sensing the Breath

Many aspects of our physical functioning can also be sensory events. Breathing is also a sensory experience if you allow yourself to focus your attention on it.

When You Are Ready

- Take each breath as you would take a sip of cool water on a thirsty day.

- From the first breath, feel the air as it passes through your nose. Is it cool or is it warm? Can you feel its fluid movement over the soft structures at the back of the throat? Notice the difference in how the air feels moving inward compared to moving outward.

- As you fill your lungs, feel the outward movement of the chest and abdomen. Do your clothes move ever so slightly against your skin?

- Sense the slight movement of your chest against your upper arms and your clothing.

- Notice how your heart rate increases slightly with each inward breath and slows again with each exhale.

- Allow yourself a moment to appreciate the perfection of the warm sensations of feeling relaxed and calm.

- Ever so gently, release this breath, allowing it to slowly flow back out. Savor each element of the experience without rushing.

- Consider each breath as a perfect refreshing moment. Although each one is perfect, there is no limit on how many perfect moments or perfect breaths we are each allowed.

- To complete the exercise, return your concentration to your breathing.

Technique 3: Slowing the Breathing

One of the hallmarks of being thoroughly relaxed is breathing at a slower rate. Conversely, one way to aid physical relaxation is to voluntarily slow the breathing.

When You Are Ready

- Without exerting any perceptible effort, slightly increase the volume of your breath. When the volume is increased, there is a tendency to exhale faster. Resist this temptation. Neither should you hold your breath in the usual fashion by closing your airway.

- Make the pause between inspiration and expiration as effortless as possible. This moment is an interlude, a peaceful episode. The beating of your heart should be your only companion in that moment.

- Feel the rhythm of your breathing, the gentle in and the gentle out. Dwell on the slow and peaceful cadence.

- Follow each in-breath and each out-breath with your attention. Occasionally open yourself to the sensations from the rest of your body.

- Savor each perfect peaceful sensation. Become a sponge to the calming physical effect of sensing your breath.

- Explore the feeling of well-being it conveys; become intimate with it.

- Reach for this feeling and reconstruct it each time you contemplate your breathing even when you are not meditating.

- Return your concentration to your breathing to complete the meditation exercise.

MINDFULNESS OF MOVEMENT

Simple activities such as walking can also be sensory experiences that can be exploited for meditation exercises. Two examples are provided in the following text. You will notice that both activities, although quite different, share a striking similarity. They are both mundane activities, things you might do every day of your life. You may ask: How can these ordinary activities be transformed into meditation? The answer to this reasonable question is this. It is not what you do in meditation, it is how you do it. If walking is nothing more than inexpensive transportation that takes too long, then it is simply walking. If you are *mindful*, that is, consciously aware of your walking, then it is meditation. If you are aware of the movements and feelings of your body, how it moves and how it breathes, you will have transcended the ordinary experience of walking. You can choose to walk to center yourself and to seek respite in your consciousness. You can choose to walk to accompany prayer and set aside the demands of the world. But this is a conscious choice of the intellect. This is meditation.

Although you may consider the following exercises novel, give them a fair try once you have mastered the basics of meditation. You may find, as have the Japanese, that even the commonplace can become an art form.

Technique 1: Walking

Walking has almost become a lost form of relaxation because we live such hurried lives. When walking was one of the few modes of transportation, it was a way of life. Today, we recognize walking as an important exercise to maintain cardiovascular health. In addition, walking helps maintain bone strength and physical stamina, as well as aiding elimination as we age. For those who do not tolerate more stressful forms of exercise, walking is only surpassed by swimming in terms of beneficial outcomes.

Like breathing, we take the skill of walking for granted almost as soon as we master it. In this exercise, each movement and intention of walking is appreciated separately and repeatedly. Walking meditation is not an issue of distance or speed, so it is not even necessary to go outside to do it. It is sufficient to be able to walk a distance of about ten steps and turn around again.

You may prepare for this exercise by performing the initial relaxation exercise in your usual position or standing, whichever you prefer. You will only need to be able to get to your feet freely and easily. In this exercise, you will need to keep your eyes open to avoid falling. You may find it helpful to direct your gaze toward your feet to maintain your concentration. The pace should be slow and deliberate, while at the same time easy and gentle. Do not walk so slowly as to lose your balance, but let your momentum carry you.

When You Are Ready

- Stand tall and erect without moving. Allow your arms to hang relaxed from your shoulders. Take a few slow, deep breaths.

- As you begin to take your first step, slowly lift your leg and foot upward. Sense the weight of your lower leg and foot.

- Swing the foot forward, making your foot the pendulum attached to your knee. Feel the momentum of the swing on your foot and lower leg.

- Place your foot gently but firmly on the ground, taking care that you do not overextend the length of your usual gait. Notice how the foot adjusts in shape to being placed on the ground. Listen for the sound of your footstep.

- Fully place the weight of your body on this foot and leg. Take into consciousness the upright position of your body, the placement of each arm, the tilt of your head and neck.

- Continue to breathe softly and easily to avoid holding your breath at any time.

- Allow the heel of the remaining foot to lift slightly and rock upward.

- Slowly and carefully lift the remaining leg and foot with the tip of the toes being last to leave the ground. Turn your attention to the bottom of your foot. Attend to the sensation apparent when the weight of the body is fully removed from this foot.

- Feel the arc of the pendulum of this foot in motion. Does one leg brush against the other? Can you hear your clothing rustle? Does your foot create the slightest movement of the air next to your other leg?

- As you place your foot ahead of the other, pay attention to how your balance changes from side to side. Feel the movement of your lower arms and hands against the outer portion of your upper legs.

- Listen to the sounds created by your clothing and movement.

- Return your attention now to your other foot and leg. Continue to work through each separate sensation and movement of walking and turning.

- Return your concentration to your breathing at any point in the process and thus complete the meditation.

NOTES: Try to maintain an even pace throughout the exercise to aid in concentration. You may also add counting from one to ten to the walking meditation exercise. This is helpful to crowd out intrusive thoughts.

Technique 2: The Tea Ceremony

Traditional oriental customs include many rituals around the preparation and serving of food. Over the centuries, the preparation and serving of tea has also been adapted as a method of meditation through a special activity or ceremony. Although the traditional ceremony includes lighting a fire to boil the water and using special dishes and utensils, we can easily adapt this model to the way we live. If you find this technique appealing, you can also select special dishes and utensils to add to the behavioral conditioning effect of regular meditation practice. It is not the precise behaviors or instruments used that make a tea ceremony a meditation. It is the deliberateness, the mindfulness, and the concentration given to what is done. This form of meditation uses an ordinary, everyday event such as the preparation of tea (or coffee or whatever) to explore the consciousness of the moment. The more mindless, unimportant, and habitual the event the better. You may choose any such activity that fits with your lifestyle. Thus, the following exercise should be used to outline the scope of this form of meditation and is not limited to the preparation of tea.

When You Are Ready

- Before beginning, take several deep and slow breaths.

- Gently pick up your empty tea kettle with your hand. Notice if the handle is cool or warm to your touch. Feel the weight of the kettle in your hand.

- Gently and easily turn to the water faucet. Place your hand on the handle while noting its temperature and texture.

- Place the kettle under the water spout and turn the water on at a moderate flow rate.

- Listen to the voice of the water falling into the kettle's empty interior. Notice how the sound changes as the water level rises.

- Watch the thousands of swarming bubbles flowing around the plunging flow of water into the kettle.

- When the kettle is filled, turn off the water and lift the kettle. Feel how much heavier the kettle is now than before.

- Turn back to the stove and place the kettle on the burner. Note the sensation of each footstep and the sound of your movements.

- Place your hand on the knob that lights and adjusts the heat. Is the surface of the knob smooth or rough, warm or cool?

- Turn on the heat under the kettle, listening for the sound made by the switch. Listen for the sound of the flame or the tapping noises of the heating element.

- Carefully attend to your breathing as the water heats. Watch for the tiny steam vapors that waft over the surface of the water before it boils and that emanate from the sides of the kettle.

- Listen for the tiniest bubbles that germinate from the sides of the kettle and rise to the water's surface. Marvel at their number and their energy while breathing softly in and out.

- To prepare for tea, open the cupboard, being mindful of reaching and stretching with your arms. Take your favorite tea cup in hand. Feel its weight and the smooth, round surface.

- Place it on the counter before you. Peer into its hollow, shiny center. Mentally rest there for a moment.

- Take in hand the tiny envelope of tea. It is so light and delicate. Carefully lift the flap of its wrapper. Listen for the faint but abrupt sounds of the paper wrapper as you peel back the flap. Under the flap you see a colored tab on the end of a string. Notice the shape, color, and texture of the paper tab crossed at an angle with a fine metal staple to hold the string.

- Let the faintest scent of the dried tea catch your attention. Allow this delicate and pleasant scent to permeate your awareness. Unhurriedly, linger in the aroma.

- Taking the tab in your hand, pull the full length of string away from the envelope. Feel the tug when you have pulled the string taut. Listen for the sound of paper against paper as the bag of tea slides from the envelope.

- Watch the tiny bag swing out and away from the envelope. See how it swings back again like the pendulum of a clock. With the other hand, grasp the tiny bag of tea leaves. Gently feel the crunchy contents between your fingers.

- Lift the bag over the opening of the tea cup. Slowly lower the bag to rest in its waiting cup. Rest your gaze and your concentration there in the cup with the tea bag.

- Turn your gaze again to your boiling kettle. Listen to the rush of the agitated water while you turn off the heat. As you reach toward the handle of the kettle, notice how warm the air becomes as your hand nears it.

- Slowly grasp the kettle's handle while avoiding the spout steam. Firmly and carefully lift the kettle over the waiting cup.

- Catch the first aroma of steaming water rushing over the tiny bag of tea. Watch how the water swirls round and round in the cup. See how the vortex pulls the tea bag with it. Notice how the boiling water has begun to darken slightly from the tea.

- Safely place the kettle back on the stove and notice how heavy the kettle is now, one cup lighter.

- Return your attention to the cup of brewing tea. After only moments, the color of the water has changed even more. You can see the essence of the tea swirling from the surface of the tiny bag containing the tea leaves.

- Breathing in the aroma of tea, gently touch the sides of the tea cup with your fingertips. The smooth surface of the cup is gingerly warm to touch. Reside in this compelling moment, pulled between desiring the first sip and fearing the heat.

- In a smooth, unhurried motion, lift the cup to your lips. Your breath disturbs and pulls at the streaks of steam that rise from the cup. With great care, gently direct your breath and blow it over the tea, causing ripples on its surface.

- Purse your mouth and take in the smallest sip of tea.

- Return your concentration to your breathing now or at any time to complete the meditation.

NOTE: You may choose to extend or shorten activity meditations like the tea ceremony at any time that is comfortable for you. The meditation exercise described here ends with the first sip of tea because the focus of the exercise is the preparation of the tea, not the drinking of it. The activity is the meditation. In the same fashion, any routine activity that holds no special connotation or negative undertone may be transformed into a meditative practice through mindful practice. In this way, the mundane portions of our lives can serve as interludes of tranquility. This is especially true if you choose to make these mindful practices a regular habit.

MINDFULNESS USING VISUALIZATION

There are several similarities between the many techniques for meditation. One such similarity is the use of the senses to achieve a thoroughly relaxed physical state. The exercises described in this section don't rely on sight as much as the ability to create vivid pictures in the imagination. These meditations work well for those who are able to fill in the visual detail of each exercise. Some of the most pleasant and satisfying meditations are those that are rich with detail. By creating these scenes in your consciousness, you effectively exclude the usual random flow of ideas that disturb contemplation.

Visualization techniques are also found in several other meditation exercises described later in this chapter. The visualization exercises that follow may also be audiotaped for actual practice. Pauses are noted in the text to guide the reader when taping for personal or group use. A pause should be as long as one complete breath (one in-breath and one out-breath). Longer pauses should be inserted between individual instructions or sets of instructions.

Technique 1: Bubbles

Following is a variation on a structured meditation described by Lawrence LeShan (1974, p. 60), which is often used in meditation classes for beginners. The purpose of this exercise is twofold. This exercise permits each thought to be acknowledged, but limits the amount of time demanded by or invested in it. Ideas or thoughts are not explored or probed, but merely recognized as thoughts. Second, the practice demonstrates how randomly thoughts appear in our consciousness. Although we may believe that our thinking is linear or connected, this is not always true. Some thoughts are spontaneous in the timing of their appearance, while others may be habitual. This exercise is one way of controlling the effect of random or distressing thoughts that create wear and tear on our health and consciousness.

When You Are Ready

- Picture yourself sitting comfortably at the bottom of a cool, clear lake. (pause) You feel relaxed and very fluid, like the water surrounding you.

- Breathe deeply and calmly several times to allow yourself to fully relax.

- In this meditative state, observe how extraneous thoughts intrude on your consciousness.

- Recognize these thoughts as intruders. (pause) Calmly and gently watch as one of these intrusive thoughts becomes encapsulated in a silvery bubble of air. (pause) The thought takes shape and immediately begins its peaceful ascent to the surface.

- Although your eyes are closed and the picture is only in your mind, every detail is sharp and clear. (pause) Notice how the bubble constantly and gently changes shape as it moves through the water. See how it weaves and darts upward at a slow and predictable pace.

- With full attention, watch this thought travel the long distance to the water's surface (which takes at least as long as two complete breaths in this resting state).

- Finally, the bubble has reached the top. (pause) You can even see the concentric ripples it causes on the surface of this cool, clear lake above you.

- Every thought that trespasses your concentration is immediately reshaped into a silvery bubble. (pause) At the instant of its transformation, it begins the wafting trip to the surface.

- Here is another intruder. (pause) How quickly it is snatched into the form of an air bubble. (pause) Quickly, it moves up and away.

- Proceed with the identification and entrapment of the intruding thoughts. Watch them become separate from you and make their way to the surface above you.

- Whenever you are ready, return your concentration to your breathing and complete the meditation.

NOTE: If this setting, the bottom of a lake, is disturbing to you, a comparable type of visual setting can be substituted with equal effect. You may choose to picture yourself sitting on the crest of a mountain or on a sandy beach. Intrusive thoughts can take the form of cliff swallows or sea birds who then wing their way out of sight into the distance. Thoughts can also become puffs of smoke that waft away on gentle breezes. Again, the purpose of this exercise is to learn how to deal with the stream of thoughts that invade your consciousness during meditation exercises. Thus, you may choose any setting and any form for your thoughts to take.

Technique 2: Basking in the Light

One of the most notable physical sensations achieved through meditation is the sensation of warmth. This exercise combines the technique of visualization with that effect. This combination is particularly satisfying to achieve deep relaxation during meditation to maintain that sense of warmth afterward.

When You Are Ready

- With your eyes closed, assume a comfortable position of your choice, preferably in a sitting position.

- Center yourself in your breathing. (pause) Follow each breath slowly in and slowly out. (pause) Dwell in each moment and in each in-breath and in each out-breath.

- In your consciousness, visualize yourself in a dark and empty space. (pause) Allow yourself to feel perfectly relaxed and comfortable in this space and at this moment.

- Directly above and in front of you, you see a tiny twinkling of light that pierces the darkness.

- This tiny ray of light now doubles in size, but shines only on you. All else is shadowed in darkness.

- This clear, bright beam again doubles in size as you begin to feel its warmth on your face and forehead. (pause) Ever so slightly, tilt your head back to catch more of its warmth on your face.

- The warmth of this light seems to flow in waves across your upper body. (pause) You begin to feel the light relax the muscles of your face while the slightest hint of a smile creeps across your lips.

- The column of light gently warms your shoulders and your arms. (pause) You turn the palms of your hands upwards to catch the warmth of the light.

- Your hands and your fingers begin to feel warm and very relaxed. (pause) You can feel the tingle of your circulation in your hands and fingers stimulated by the light.

- You peacefully and gently dwell in this circle of light. (pause) The waves of gentle relaxation continue to wash down your body from your face and head, (pause) now to your shoulders, (pause) now to your upper arms, (pause) and now all the way to your hands and fingers.

- Whenever you are ready to complete the meditation, simply return your concentration to your breathing.

MINDFULNESS IN REFLECTION

Reflection is a different type of meditation exercise than those already presented. Reflective meditations are opportunities to deliberately and mentally explore a particular subject. As an example of this technique, the following exercise is presented to explore a concept important to nurses and to nursing; that is, compassion. The following meditation follows the model of reflective meditation and is designed to serve as an example of other meditations that can be developed at the option of the reader.

Meditation on Compassion

In the vernacular of nurses, compassion is the ability to commiserate with our patients without pitying them. Compassionate nurses are not indifferent to the suffering of their patients; they are empathetic with them. Empathy differs from sympathy in that empathy is the ability to personally identify with the suffering and pain. Sympathy is feeling sorry for another person. The critical difference in nursing's view is that sympathetic caring will undermine nursing's efforts to help patients care for themselves and remain independent. If we only feel sorry for our patients, then we may do things for them that they should do for themselves. Empathetic nursing care, on the other hand, is directed toward making patients and their families independent decision makers and caregivers. The empathetic nurse recognizes, first and foremost, that the primary role of the nurse is that of an advocate, rather than a servant or best friend, for patients.

When You Are Ready

- Make yourself comfortable in whatever position suits you best to remain attentive throughout the exercise. (pause) Go slowly through each step of the relaxation process and avoid rushing yourself.

- Center yourself by taking great care to concentrate on your breathing. (pause) Experience the physical sensations of each breath. (pause) Drink in each breath, slowly in and slowly out.

- While in this deep, relaxed state, think about all of the patients and families you have encountered over your time in nursing, no matter how short.

- Think back and remember, did you ever have a patient or family member that made you angry? (pause) What did he do to make you angry? (pause) What did you do in return? (pause) How has this experience changed the way you treat your patients and their families now?

- Did a patient or a family member ever physically hurt you? (pause) What did she do to injure you? (pause) What did you do in return? (pause) How has this experience changed the way you treat your patients and their families now?

- Did a patient or family member ever hurt your feelings? (pause) What did they do to hurt your feelings? (pause) What did you do in return? (pause) How has this experience changed the way you treat your patients and their families now?

- Have you ever made one of your patients angry? (pause) Have you ever caused one of your patients undue pain or discomfort? (pause) Have you ever caused hurt feelings in one of your patients? (pause) How have these experiences changed the way you treat your patients and their families now?

- Did you ever have a patient that reminded you of yourself, that you personally identified with? (pause) What was it about him that made you personally identify with him?

- Mentally change places with this person for just one second. (pause) How does this make you feel about this person? (pause) What makes him angry or sad or hurts his feelings? (pause) What makes you angry or sad or hurts your feelings?

- What will you do differently to better care for your patients and their families? (pause)

MANTRA MEDITATION TECHNIQUES

One of the peculiar stereotypes many people carry around about meditation surrounds the use of mantras. When meditation was popularized by Maharishi Mahesh Yogi, one of the hallmarks of meditating was having a special word or sound to use repeatedly to block out errant thoughts. When meditation lessons were given, each student was given a special word-sound that was to remain a secret only known to the student. Frequently, the mantra used was the word *Om*, which is a Sanskrit word for God. Many people thought mantras were quite a novelty and the popular media frequently capitalized on the unusual idea of a person incessantly repeating the same word over and over. Although the media made light of the practice, the use of a mantra is not unlike the litanies, the repetition of The Lord's Prayer or the Amidah found in Christian churches and synagogues.

A mantra can be any word, sound, or simple prayer; the choice is up to the individual. The way the mantra is used is very similar to the breathing exercises described earlier in this chapter. The meditation exercise should begin by systematically relaxing the whole body. Once you are totally relaxed, the mantra is repeated silently or whispered slowly and deliberately. One rationale for the constant repetition is to exclude rambling thoughts

from intruding into the meditative interlude. Mantras are frequently simple sounds, rather than a particular word. This is to
avoid generating thoughts based on whatever ideas a particular
word may evoke. Some people prefer to use a word like *Amen,*
which is both devotional and has a positive feeling to it.

When You Are Ready

- Take all the time you need to become fully relaxed.

- Center yourself in your breathing. Come back to it at
  any time during the meditation period to recenter yourself.

- Softly and gently repeat the mantra to yourself. Use
  your mantra with your breathing to set up a smooth
  and easy rhythm.

- Concentrate on your mantra and the cycles of repetition.
  If outside thoughts intrude, refocus yourself on your
  breathing and then on your mantra.

- When you have completed your meditation period,
  return to your breathing and thus complete your meditation exercise.

GUIDED MINDFULNESS AND GUIDED MEDITATIONS

The meditations to follow are different from those already
described. The previous meditations should be reviewed before
meditating to give inexperienced persons a full description of
how to proceed on their own. It is not important that the exact
sequence of events be followed or to memorize the exact words
used in each description. The following meditations differ in
that the person meditating is guided through the process by
another person or by an audiotape. Each meditation focuses on
a particular emotional challenge. Although there are many similarities between all of the exercises listed, these exercises work
best if they are read aloud to the person (or group) who is
meditating. You can tape these meditations yourself for your

own use or record them for others to be played back during their meditation exercises.

Because everyone's needs are different in relation to the topics covered in the guided meditation, permit the person who is to meditate to review the text of the meditation before actually using the meditation. Some people who are in the process of grieving the loss of a loved one may not feel comfortable with the meditation on dealing with grief. They may feel more comfortable with the meditation on releasing first because it is more general in nature and emotionally less threatening. The same may be true for the meditation for survivors of abuse. Releasing feelings of hurt and extreme emotion has a cleansing value. Many people have not been able to work through and heal after various traumas because the emotional component is still too strong. The releasing meditation is recommended as a good starting place for those who carry physical or emotional distress. Remember that the key to using all the exercises is to be sufficiently prepared by becoming fully relaxed mentally and physically.

The benefit of repeated use of a releasing meditation cannot be overemphasized. Although some experiences have truly been painful, the sufferer needs to be completely willing to let go of the pain. This may seem to be a curious point. However, the sufferer must examine what purpose the experience has served in her emotional and spiritual consciousness. If this purpose has not yet been recognized or acknowledged, the emotional attachment to it may be too strong. The lesson must often be practiced over and over until it is mastered. This mastery takes time and cannot be hurried.

The final point to be made in these introductory comments is that the following exercises were designed with the same purpose. This purpose is to allow the individual to transcend these various intrapersonal challenges. Death, pain, and grief are inevitable aspects of the human experience. On the most superficial level, all humans have to face the reality of these difficult experiences at some time. Meditation can be useful to desensitize and destress these experiences. On a higher level, we must also learn to cope with and surpass these experiences. We do not have the luxury of ignoring or avoiding these inevitable experiences. Meditation can provide a safe environment to encounter these challenges and overcome the emotional restrictions they may place on our daily lives. We must survive. Internally, we must find the courage and strength to shake off the emotional envelope that surrounds these challenges. As a fellow human being, you face the same fate as your patients. As a health care provider, you may be called upon to support the patient or the family during these times of great stress. However, what happens when the pain is yours? What happens when you, the nurse, are not available, or when the family and patient go home? Meditation is the sort of therapy that can be self-applied *prn ad lib* with confidence and caring.

Guided Meditation: Releasing

There are many challenges in our daily lives. We frequently meet challenges that we cannot master or overcome. As frustration builds, we tend to escalate our effort and work even harder to fix the problem. These problems may be things, conditions, our health, our jobs, our loved ones, or even a poor choice we have made. However, there comes a point where no amount of effort on our part will change what is, what has been, or what will be. When we reach this point in our struggle, we are usually exhausted mentally and physically. The Eastern cultures speak eloquently to resolving this type of problem. They instruct us to cease to struggle against the problem. Stop trying to change our loved ones. Stop resisting the situation. The following meditation is an exercise to that end. You may read this meditation to yourself silently or aloud, or you may read it to someone else.

When You Are Ready

- Assume a comfortable position that will also allow attentiveness throughout the exercise. (pause) Go slowly through the process and avoid rushing any step.
- Work through the steps to relax the body systematically and completely using your breathing.
- Center yourself in your breathing. (pause) Experience your body and your breathing in the present moment.

(pause) Allow yourself to drift on each breath you take. Slowly in and slowly out, thoroughly relaxed.

- While in this deep relaxed state, visualize a natural pool of clear blue water surrounded by lush green ferns and almost overgrown with fernlike trees.

- Looking down into the water, you can even see the small pebbles lying deep below the water. The water is peaceful and quiet.

- There are the tiniest ripples on the surface. These tiny waves move silently toward the far edge just out of sight.

- Now you can barely hear the sound of the tiny ripples flowing out of the pool through the trees beyond.

- A leaf from an overhanging tree floats gently onto the surface of the water almost within your reach.

- The soft, green leaf lingers there, floating on the mirrored surface. It does not sink, but drifts like a fragile boat.

- Almost imperceptibly, the leaf begins to glide uncertainly toward the far side of the pool. You admire how gently and peacefully the leaf makes its way to the tiny waterfall on the far side.

- Suddenly the leaf disappears over the edge out of sight. You cannot see the leaf, but again you hear the ripple of flowing water.

- You breathe in the peace and quiet, resting quietly in its beauty.

- In this calm and relaxed state, you mentally reach into your pocket and take out a small piece of paper and a small pencil.

- You have had something on your mind recently that has worried you greatly. You are here at the water's edge because you are ready to release this worry from your consciousness.

- In a word or two, you write the nature of this problem on the small slip of paper.

- Having done so, you slowly put the pencil back in your pocket and hold the piece of paper at arm's length over the pool of silent water. (pause)

- Breathing deeply, you affirm to yourself that the outcome of this worry or problem will be for the better. In doing so, you also forgive yourself for any role you have played in the problem and forgive any other person for his role in the problem.

- You also release any anger or frustration over this problem as you prepare to release this problem from your consciousness and the paper from your grip. Like a slow motion film, you clearly see your fingers open wide and the tiny slip of paper dip and dive down out of your grip.

- The note looks like it barely touches the water and circles there peacefully for a moment.

- The words you wrote on the paper are already wet as the paper takes the route of the leaf to the pool's far edge.

- You breathe deeply and calmly, watching this problem detach itself from you and move away. You also detach yourself from the emotions surrounding this problem. There is no more struggle, no more frustration.

- Suddenly the note is gone, having slipped out of the pool down behind the trees.

- Again you can barely hear the murmur of softly falling water.

- The relief from the burden is evident on your face. You carry a smile of affection and peace, a gentle smile.

- You breathe deeply and remind yourself that this peaceful place is always here for you. You can return at will and bring other problems to the water's edge. (pause) The water is there for your refreshment.

- When you are ready to finish, return your concentration to your breathing and thus complete the meditation.

Guided Meditation: On Pain

For many people, especially nurses, the relief of pain means the administration of drugs. A good nurse knows all the brand names, dosages, methods of delivery, and just when and how to administer them for the best result. But we have all cared for patients who are experiencing, or experienced ourselves, unrelenting or intractable pain. Sometimes, we have patients who cannot tolerate the drugs we have to offer due to allergies or side effects. Nothing is quite as frustrating as trying to manage pain with all the expertise we have and yet be unsuccessful.

It is important to remember that pain is a subjective experience. We learn to interpret pain according to our previous experiences with it. As young children, we first discover pain when we are learning to walk and fall, scraping our knees or bumping our heads. In our mind's eye, pain becomes associated with failure, making mistakes, and error. Thus, we all sincerely believe that pain is bad and should be avoided at all costs. However, pain plays an important role in the diagnostic and treatment process. The location, character, and duration of pain is vital information in the identification of disease processes and a valid indicator of treatment effectiveness.

We all know that the pain that arises from some conditions cannot be totally eliminated. Chronic conditions such as arthritis demand a pain management routine that can be maintained for the balance of a lifetime. Meditation can be an important adjunct to all other therapies. It can be used consistently without fear of untoward side effects.

When You Are Ready

- Assume a comfortable position that will also allow attentiveness throughout the exercise. (pause) Go slowly through the process and avoid rushing any step.

- Work through the steps to relax the body systematically and completely using your breathing.

- Center yourself in your breathing. (pause) Experience your body and your breathing in the present moment, both the painful sensations and the warm, pleasant ones.

- Turn your consciousness to the pain. (pause) What are the sensations that make up the pain message? (pause) Is the pain message steady or intermittent? (pause) What is the nature of the pain?

- What is the pain message? (pause) Are there emotions tied to the pain message? (pause) Recognize those messages, the anger, fear, or anxiety.

- Breathe with the sensations of the pain message. (pause) Become mindful of the physical and emotional aspects of this sensation called pain.

- Visualize your breath moving through the body part where the pain arises. (pause) Visualize each calm and peaceful breath flowing through the pain.

- Recognize that the pain sensation is only a sensation and nothing else. (pause) The pain is not part of your identity and you do not own this pain. (pause) You are merely experiencing pain at this time.

- Accept the pain as an aspect of this present moment. (pause) Do not react to the pain or judge it.

- Distance yourself from the sensations of the pain experience. (pause) Release any emotional interpretations you have about your pain.

- Dwell in the moment of the experience. (pause) Just be present here and now.

- Use your breathing to massage and destress the pain experience.

- You may return your concentration to your breathing at any time, thus completing the meditation.

Guided Meditation: Working Through Grief

Grief is a natural response to loss. The losses that we experience can be very significant, such as the death of a loved one, or much less important, such as the loss of a family pet. Grief can also be felt in anticipation of an expected loss. Many people experience anticipatory grief when a loved one has an aggressively debilitating condition. The sense of loss can be as acute before the loved one's death as afterward. Grief of this type frequently marks the involuntary end of one lifestyle and the mandatory beginning of another. Wives become widows, husbands become widowers, parents become childless, and children become orphans. For many, the feeling of grief is focused on the loss of someone who was a lifelong companion and friend. Sometimes this person is a spouse or a grown child, or perhaps a sibling. The grief they feel is the loss of the presence of that special person in their life. This emptiness is a void that cannot be filled by simply making new friends or staying occupied.

A meditation exercise like the following example is one way to offer some consolation and solace for either anticipatory grieving or grieving the death of a loved one. This exercise is designed to allow the person meditating to reconnect with the positive energies and feelings surrounding the positive memories of that special person. Keep in mind that this is not a mystical exercise that purports to raise spirits from the dead. This meditation is, however, an exercise in remembering the good feelings of being with that special person. It is also an exercise in remembering the special person as she was in health and wellness. It is an exercise in gaining perspective: forgetting the more recent memories of suffering and remembering when times were better. Be mindful that this exercise is not designed as a one-dose therapy. Working through grief takes time to resolve and tears may be shed in the process. This meditation is an exercise that will bear repeating many times to gradually work through the loss of a loved one.

When You Are Ready

- Assume a comfortable position that will also allow you to be attentive, yet relaxed, throughout this exercise.

- Center yourself in your breathing. (pause) Experience the sensations of your body and your breathing in the present moment. With each in-breath and each out-breath, let yourself experience each pleasant and peaceful sensation.

- Totally focus on your breathing. (pause) There is no past moment or future moments, only the present moment. (pause) Dwell in the sensations of how you feel right now, so calm and peaceful.

- In your mind's eye, see yourself in a warm, sunlit room where time cannot intrude. You are calm and everything is at peace. (pause) As you breathe deeply, you feel a great sense of well-being. (pause) Experience every in-breath and every out-breath as a new experience.

- While resting in this timeless room, full of peace and warmth, thoughts of a special person come to mind. This special person is no longer with you now in the physical sense, because he has passed on. (pause) However, in your mind, you bring all of your good thoughts and favorite memories of this special person into this warm and peaceful room with you.

- In your mind's eye, you see yourself and this special person sitting together, quietly enjoying the company of each other in this wonderful place. (pause) You have no need for words. You are both very calm and everything is at peace.

- Again when you breathe deeply, you both feel a great sense of well-being by being here together in the endless present moment. (long pause)

- While you abide together in this quiet place, there is no pain or suffering permitted here. (pause) There is only peace and calm.

- As you abide together in this quiet place, there is no fear or grief. (pause) There is only peace and love. (long pause)

- You dwell in this peaceful place together until you and your special person are completely saturated with the company of each other. (long pause)

- Having shared this time with your special person in your consciousness, remember that this place always exists for you to recall this special person. (pause)

- When you are satisfied, you can bring your consciousness back to your breathing. Even in doing so, you
retain that feeling of warmth and comfort from remembering your special person. Let this feeling linger. Hold
on to it. Make it last.

Guided Meditation: Forgiveness

Without exception, every nurse has encountered someone who
has an emotional problem. Emotional problems can take many
forms. In particular, guilt can be an emotional problem that can
exacerbate or inflate other physical symptoms of stress. Guilt is
a peculiar problem in that many people can feel guilty for events
over which they had no control. Although the legal definition of
guilt is tied to harmful intention, the emotional aspects of guilt are
not. Parents may feel guilt if they have a child born with a congenital deformity. Children may feel guilty if their parents choose
to divorce. Survivors of abuse often feel guilty that they somehow
brought the abuse upon themselves; that they somehow deserved
to be abused. Intellectually, we all know the difference between
innocence and guilt, but our emotional side is much more vulnerable to confusion. Emotions are much more complex and frequently demand readjustment or healing.

One of the first steps to begin the emotional healing from
guilt is to work with self-forgiveness. Many people find it easy to
forgive others, but find it hard to forgive themselves. Like the previous meditation on grieving, the following exercise is designed
to dissipate guilt and clarify the balance between guilt and forgiveness. Again, this exercise may be repeated as necessary to
work through healing. Remember, healing is a process and one
meditation is only the equivalent of one small treatment. The
more serious the wound, the more treatments that are needed.
The same premise is also applied to problems like grieving or
feelings of guilt.

When You Are Ready

- Assume a comfortable position that will also permit you
to be attentive throughout the exercise. (pause) Go
slowly and avoid rushing any step.

- Center yourself in your breathing. (pause) Experience your body and your breathing in the present moment in complete relaxation.

- When you are fully centered, you are completely safe and secure. (pause) You are fully insulated from the outside world, yet perfectly free and safe.

- While in this safe and secure place, envision the person you love most in the universe. This person can be anyone you love the most, a person who is living or dead. In your mind's eye, envision your loved one healthy and happy and whole.

- Now take a minute to smile to yourself and enjoy the mental presence of your loved one. (pause) Remember all of the good things about this person and the love you feel for her. (pause) Hold those good thoughts.

- Do you remember the good times laughing and talking with this person? Does it make you smile again? Do you remember the sound of her voice, her funny expressions? (pause) Hold those good feelings.

- Right now, experience how your body feels when you think about this person you love most in the universe. (pause) Do you feel warm and happy? Can you feel the smile on your own face? (pause) Feel on the inside what it is you are feeling on the outside.

- With this vision of your loved one in your mind's eye, ask yourself a question. What if something very bad happened because this person made a bad decision or made a mistake. Would you forgive her for what had happened? (pause) Of course you would forgive the person you love most in the universe. She deserves your love and forgiveness, doesn't she?

- What does that forgiveness feel like to your body? (pause) How does forgiveness feel inside of you? (pause) Think about your loved one and experience this feeling of forgiving. (pause) In the silence of your heart, speak words of loving forgiveness to your loved one.

- Forgiveness erases the pain and distress. (pause) Afterwards, there is no more guilt to forgive.

- Center yourself again in your breathing. (pause) Experience again this safe and secure space in your consciousness.

- Now turn your conscious focus to yourself. In your own heart, answer this question: Have you ever felt guilty because something bad happened to you, or you made a bad decision, or you made a mistake? (pause) How does this guilt feel to your body?

- Although you may have carried this guilt with you for a long time, think how quickly you were ready to forgive the person you loved most in the universe. (pause) In your mind's eye, mentally see yourself as that person you love most in the universe. Just as you did before, go through the experience of feeling forgiveness and being forgiven.

- In the silence of your heart, speak words of loving forgiveness to yourself. (pause) What does that forgiveness feel like to your body? (pause) How does forgiveness feel inside of you? (pause) Think about yourself and experience this feeling of forgiving and forgiveness.

- Forgiveness erases the guilt and the pain and the distress. (pause) Afterwards, there is no more guilt to forgive. You are forgiven. You are completely forgiven. Feel the forgiveness.

- Center yourself again in your breathing. (pause) Experience again this safe and secure place in your consciousness. (pause) Remember, you can return to this place whenever you desire. This place is a well of peace and forgiveness. Come and drink from it any time you desire.

- You may return your concentration to your breathing at any time and thus complete the meditation.

SUMMARY

The exercises included in this chapter have been designed as samples and examples of various types of meditations. There are many fine books and audiotapes on meditation that can be found in public libraries and bookstores everywhere. These books and tapes are just like any other consumer product; some are more appealing than others. If you are a nurse who would like to begin meditating regularly, shop around until you find something that suits you. If you are a nurse who is interested in teaching meditation to your patients, do the same. Shop around until you find a variety of materials that suits your patient population. Consider the age and backgrounds of your patients. If they are predominantly Catholic, then shop the Catholic bookstores. If they are Jewish, visit the bookstore at the synagogue, and so on. Feel free to adapt the examples included in this text to fit the language styles and level of understanding of your patients. You don't even have to use the word *meditation* if you feel that using a term like *centering exercises* may be more appropriate. In any case, apply these exercises as you would any nursing therapy, knowing that the best kind of treatment is one that has been individualized for that very patient.

As was mentioned before, the meditations included in chapters 5 and 6 are included as clip-out exercises in the appendix. If the reader wishes to use these exercises for group activities, it will be necessary to help the group become relaxed initially and then to end the meditation in like fashion. The group leader should be mindful that these processes take time and cannot be rushed. A good meditation session can be thwarted if the relaxation is interrupted by closure that comes too suddenly. If you are new to leading meditation activities, then you will need to prepare an appropriate lead-in to some of the clip-out exercises and/or a suitable conclusion for some of them.

References

LeShan, L. (1974). *How to meditate: A guide to self-discovery.* New York: Bantam.

Merton, T. (1955). *No man is an island.* New York: Harcourt Brace.

Walshe, M. O'C. (translator). (1979). *Meister Eckhart: Sermons and treatises.* New York: Watkins.

Suggested Reading

Chopra, D. (1989). *Quantum healing: Exploring the frontiers of mind/body medicine.* New York: Bantam.

Dossey, B. M., Keegan, L., Kolkmeier, L. G., & Guzzetta, C. E. (1989). *Holistic health promotion: A guide for practice.* Rockville, MD: Aspen Publishers.

Dossey, L. (1993). *Healing words.* San Francisco: Harper.

Goldstein, J., & Kornfield, J. (1987). *Seeking the heart of wisdom: The path of insight meditation.* Boston: Shambhala.

James, W. (1982). *Varieties of religious experience: A study in human nature.* New York: Penguin.

Kabat-Zinn, J. (1990). *Full catastrophe living: Using the wisdom of your body and mind to face stress, pain, and illness.* New York: Delta.

Levine, S. (1979). *A gradual awakening.* Garden City, NY: Anchor Books.

Levine, S. (1982). *Who dies: An investigation of conscious living and conscious dying.* New York: Anchor Books.

Moore, T. (1994). *Meditations: On the monk who dwells in daily life.* New York: HarperCollins Publishers.

Nhat Hanh, T. (1975). *The miracle of mindfulness: A manual on meditation.* Boston: Beacon Press.

Norris, G. (1991). *Being home: A book of meditations.* New York: Bell Tower.

Suzuki, S. (1970). *Zen mind, beginners mind: Informal talks on Zen meditation and practice.* New York: Weatherhill.

Trungpa, C. (1969). *Meditation in action.* Boulder: Shambhala.

A

ANNOTATED
BIBLIOGRAPHY—
SELECTED WORKS

INTRODUCTORY TEXTS ON MEDITATION

Benson, H. (1976). *The relaxation response.* New York: Avon. (paperback)

This little text should be a mandatory reading assignment for every nursing student entering nursing school and should be read again in graduate programs. It is considered one of the foundational works in the area of stress and stress reduction. The discussion includes a careful and simple explanation of the effect of stress on the body and the effect of meditation on the body. Although the evidence presented in this book would seem insufficient by today's standard of scientific argument, this work has since been upheld by many investigators and by virtually every practitioner that has ever instructed a patient to take a deep breath.

Probably the most revolutionary aspect of Benson's message was that the body could be deliberately conditioned to relax, just as it could be inadvertently conditioned to become overly alert. The notion that involuntary bodily functions could be controlled in some voluntary fashion was still new to the scientific community. Today, biofeedback is widely used by specialists to treat such diverse conditions as headaches and urinary incontinence. However, it is interesting that the use of meditation by non-specialists, like the general population of nurses, is only now building impetus.

Hewitt, J. (1978). *Teach yourself meditation.* Chicago: Hodder & Stoughton.

One of many books in the Teach Yourself series, this volume is a compendium and survey of methods, including Indian Yoga, Buddhist (Tibetan, Zen, and Chinese), and Sufism. The book is well laid out and includes a full description of techniques to facilitate awareness of breathing. Visual and listening meditations are presented along with exercises designed to take the reader past psycho-physical relaxation alone.

The portion of the book that addresses these techniques aimed at heightened self awareness (Chapter 8—Who (or What) Am I? The Onion Game) is particularly noteworthy. The author clearly demonstrates the philosophical roots, Eastern and Western, common to meditative practice as a means to enlightenment beyond the ego and the physical self. The Onion Game is described as follows:

> It is a solitary quest that takes awareness beyond the clamour, clutter, and confusion of the ego into the clear space and white light of pure consciousness. . . . To dissolve the ego is not annihilation or surrender to nihilism, masters of the meditation tell us, but the discovery of the self beyond the ego. (p. 122)

In this chapter and others that follow, the author has carefully annotated his discussion with references to and quotes from a rich variety of literary sources. In doing so, the reader is tempted to further explore the works of Allan Watts, Wei Wu Wei, William James, and Aubrey Menen, as well as the historic Bhagavad Gita and the Upanishads. These discussions provide an important spiritual context to the meditative exercises described in the text. Thus, the reader is free to retrace and explore the ideas of many insightful thinkers and these important religious texts.

Ram Dass. (1990). *Journey of awakening: A meditator's guidebook* (rev. ed.). New York: Bantam Books.

This author, born Richard Alper in Boston, MA, was a psychologist in the Social Relations Department at Harvard University during the 1960s. He changed his name after finding a new spiritual direction in the meditative religious practices of

India. As a result, he has produced this text (originally published in 1978) and several others which have provided the foundation for many Westerners to understand and employ Eastern meditative practices. This text provides a complete discussion of numerous meditation techniques, as well as advice on finding support for continued growth in meditation through groups, teachers, and retreats. The reader is impressed with these discussions which convey the writer's own personal difficulties in choosing and maintaining personal growth through meditation.

One of the most valuable aspects of the book is the list of groups and centers that teach meditation or provide retreats in the United States and Canada. Although the list may not be entirely accurate at this time, it includes addresses and phone numbers, and in some cases, information about the nature of the services provided, whether religious based, monastic, or eclectic. Serious students of meditation will find this paperback book a valuable addition to their library of readings on meditation.

MEDITATION AND HEALTH CARE

Achterberg, J. (1985). *Imagery in healing: Shamanism and modern medicine.* Boston: New Science Library.

Although the major focus of this book centers on the importance of therapeutic images in the healing process, meditation is frequently presented as a vehicle to convey these healing energies. Nurse readers will also find this book important to further clarify their historical therapeutic role in the healing process.

Chopra, D. (1989). *Quantum healing: Exploring the frontiers of mind/body medicine.* New York: Bantam Books.

Dr. Chopra was born in India and has practiced endocrinology in the United States. He is the founding president of the American Association of Ayurvedic Medicine.

This book and the others Dr. Chopra has authored, including *Unconditional Life, Perfect Health,* and *Creating Health,* artfully elaborate on the principles of ancient Indian medicine (Ayurveda) and describe how to intertwine them with modern

Western medicine. Chopra's discussion employs many of the principles of quantum physics and applies them to the functioning of the body and the mind. In doing so, Chopra also describes how the mind can directly influence the body to create disease or to recreate health. With this perspective, the aim of meditation is not focused simply on Benson's relaxation response, but describes meditation as a pathway to alter consciousness and to effect healing. Numerous examples of the mind/body connection in disease and recovery are provided to illustrate this point. Again, most of the conditions described are stress related, such as cardiovascular conditions or immunologic disorders like cancer. Chopra asserts that these powerful techniques from the Ayurvedic traditions will gradually be incorporated into Western medical practices. When joined it will

> . . . create a new medicine, one of knowledge and compassion. At its best, current medicine already contains these ingredients—the medical system is in trouble, but its woes are transcended by caring individuals. They will be the first to see that Ayurveda is not in conflict with their work as doctors; it can only help the process of recovery and bring healing under our control. (p. 255)

Kabat-Zinn, J. (1990). *Full catastrophe living: Using the wisdom of your body and mind to face stress, pain, and illness.* New York: Delta.

This text describes the treatment program of the Stress Reduction Clinic at the University of Massachusetts Medical Center which was founded and is directed by Dr. Kabat-Zinn, PhD. The complete clinical program for stress reduction and chronic pain management is depicted through numerous case studies. This book will be very helpful to health care providers who wish to develop similar programs in their own settings. This clinical treatment program relies heavily on the practice of meditation to achieve physical relaxation and to permit patients to consciously alter the way in which they perceive and appraise stress.

Kabat-Zinn is careful to qualify the healing effect of meditation described as a result of this treatment program that relies heavily on meditative practice. He asserts that:

. . . there are few if any outright cures for chronic diseases or for stress-related disorders. . . . Healing implies the possibility of us to relate differently to illness, disability, even death as we learn to see with eyes of wholeness. As we have seen, this comes from practicing such basic skills as going into and dwelling in states of deep physiological relaxation and seeing and transcending our fears and our boundaries of body and mind. (p. 173)

Levine, S. (1982). *Who dies?: An investigation of conscious living and conscious dying.* New York: Doubleday.

This work examines some of the least discussed issues of death such as finishing business, dying children, suicide, funerals and working with pain. Although most health care providers frequently encounter death in their practices, literature on the therapeutic aspects of these topics is very rare. This text is presented as a mixture of contemplative readings interspersed with guided meditations that can be read silently or aloud to others. This unusual work provides an articulate and therapeutic foundation for using meditation with patients and families who are facing end-of-life challenges. Nurses who work in hospice settings will find this book an important resource to integrating meditation and nursing practice.

Moyers, B. (1993). *Healing and the mind.* New York: Doubleday.

This book was compiled to accompany a Public Broadcasting Service (PBS) series that explored the connection between the mind and healing physical disorders. As such, it features many well-known health care professionals such as Dean Ornish, MD, author of *Dr. Dean Ornish's Program for Reversing Heart Disease* and Director of the Preventive Medicine Research Institutes at the University of California, San Francisco, and Jon Kabat-Zinn, PhD, author of *Full Catastrophe Living: Using the Wisdom of Your Body and Mind to Face Stress, Pain and Illness* and Director of the Stress Reduction Clinic at the University of Massachusetts Medical Center.

This book provides an informative overview of how the practice of medicine has been slowly changing from the strictly reductionistic model of medicine where each specialty was concerned with a single organ system. Health care today is moving back to viewing the person as a whole and examining the internal and external factors that contribute to wellness and illness. As an interesting complement to the discussion, the text is punctuated with black and white, and color photographs of how contemporary and historic artists depict the human body, illness, and health care.

Pelletier, K. R. (1977). *Mind as healer, mind as slayer.* New York: Delta.

This text was first published in 1977 and is now viewed as one of the foundational works in describing the mind-body connection. The most recent printing of this book now contains a preface written in 1992 which includes a discussion of two new medical specialties that have been developed in the interim: behavioral medicine and psychoneuroimmunology. It is only fitting that an author who has contributed to the development of these new fields has now included a discussion of the advances from these areas in his text.

Along with biofeedback and autogenic training, meditation is one of the suggested methods for controlling stress. Although no exercises are included in the text, the argument for regular meditation is very compelling.

Another point to bear in mind is that there is an attitudinal component to meditation that may have a great deal to do with its success or lack thereof for a particular individual. Those who meditate have chosen to do so. (p. 194)

Siegel, B. S. (1986). *Love, medicine & miracles: Lessons learned about self-healing from a surgeon's experience with exceptional patients.* New York: Harper & Row Publishers.

Dr. Siegel is considered one of the pioneers in using individual and group therapy to treat cancer patients. At the time, he presented a new persona for health care providers who were previously portrayed as distant and aloof from patients. His work has served to suppress this dysfunctional practice and has heightened the awareness of both patients and providers about their synergistic roles in the healing process.

Weil, A. (1985). *Health and healing.* Boston: Houghton Mifflin Company.

    This book is an in-depth review of the allopathic tradition of modern medicine as well as a brief summary of alternative therapeutic choices such as osteopathy, chiropractic, naturopathy, Chinese medicine, and homeopathy. Weil provides this review to clarify to the reader the commonality in these disparate therapeutic models—the interplay between the mind and the body. The nature of placebo as a form of active or passive treatment is discussed at length. The final chapters of the book describe how allopathic medicine and what we call modern science will come to integrate this revelation about the nature of disease and the wholeness of the person (i.e., mind and body) in the next century.

    For those health professionals who have received most of their training in the allopathic tradition, which includes nurses, this book will clarify the distinctions between the limitations of traditional medical practice and the holistic perspective that nursing is purported to employ. Reading this text also reinforces the unique identity of nursing in the health care arena and the importance of providing therapies such as meditation for patients. Thus, this book is highly recommended as a conceptual foundation for today's changing health care philosophy away from acute care to preventive and holistic health care services.

EXPANDED CONSCIOUSNESS AND THE NEW PHYSICS

Bentov, I. (1977), *Stalking the wild pendulum: On the mechanics of consciousness.* Rochester, VT: Destiny Books.

    The author was an inventor without formal degrees who died in 1979. Surprisingly, he wrote this interesting book which describes the integration of what may seem diverse concepts from cosmology's big bang theory, the quantum physics of light and sound, and medicine. Like other scientist authors, Bentov presents a scientific logic that describes the mind-body connection using principles from quantum physics.

Zukav, G. (1979). *The dancing Wu Li masters: An overview of the new physics.* New York: Bantam Books.

During the early 1980s, this book was on the reading list for nursing theory courses taught by Martha Rogers. Although she had formulated her theory which described increasing resonance, increasing complexity, and energy fields many years earlier, she indicated that her theory was congruent with this field of "new physics." This book is more extensive in its discussion than that of Bentov but is characteristic of the trend in science for theories to be postulated on the cosmic scale and the human scale by studying elements at the subatomic level.

MEDITATION IN THE CONTEXT OF RELIGION

Kaplan, A. (1985). *Jewish meditation: A practical guide.* New York: Schocken Books.

In his introductory comments, this author immediately addresses the common misconception that the practice of Judaism does not include meditation. Kaplan argues that although the Judaic esoteric mystic traditions such as the Kabbalah were commonly known to employ meditation, meditation is also valid in mainstream practice. This author's earlier work, *Meditation and the Bible* (1978), is said to be derived from original translations from Hebrew which provided new descriptions of Jewish meditative practices. The actual text that follows is presented with terms and spelling in Hebrew plus numerous references to commonly used Jewish prayers.

In all, this small book is an excellent resource for professionals who work with patient populations that are predominantly Jewish. In addition, the student of meditation will also find that Kaplan provides an enlightening and rich view of meditation in the pre-Christian tradition.

Keating, T. (1994). *Open mind, open heart: The contemplative dimension of the Gospel.* New York: Continuum.

This basic text describes religious contemplation, including a detailed history of contemplative prayer from early Christianity. This author, also a monastic, emphasizes the spiritual aspects of contemplation and deemphasizes any physical effects of meditative practices. However, the appendices describe in detail the method of "Centering Prayer," which includes a helpful description of proper body positioning, the use of a mantra, or "sacred word," and techniques to refocus concentration during contemplative activities.

Kornfield, J. (1993). *A path with heart: A guide through the perils and promises of spiritual life.* New York: Bantam Books.
This book is a compilation of meditations written by an American who became a Theravada Buddhist monk. Included are many wonderful discussions and meditations: Transforming Sorrow into Compassion, Forgiveness, Reflecting on Difficulty, and Reflecting on the Cycles of Your Spiritual Life. This is the type of book that cannot be consumed all at once. It is meant to be savored and revisited.

Merton, T. (1961). *New seeds of contemplation.* New York: A New Directions Book.
Although a monastic, Merton was a prolific writer who published extensively and was acclaimed widely before his death in 1968. This text was originally published in 1962 and has been reprinted more than twenty times. His work is viewed as a mainstay in the Roman Catholic tradition of meditation in the classical religious sense.

Merton, T. (1973). *Contemplation in a world of action.* Garden City, NY: Image Books.
This was one of the very last manuscripts written by Merton. It includes insightful meditative essays on a life of contemplation in the eremetic tradition.

Mullin, G. H. (1981). *Selected works of the Dalai Lama I: Bridging the sutras and the tantras.* Ithaca, NY: Snow Lion Publications.
Translated from Tibetan, these are the most well-known works of the first Dalai Lama, Gen-dun Drub (1391–1474). These writings are said to have set the style, pace, and flavor for Buddhist writings. The chapter entitled "Notes on Training the Mind" provides a glimpse of Buddhist meditation practices as a pathway to awareness and spiritual enlightenment.

Nhat Hanh, T. (1990). *Transformation & healing: Sutra on the four establishments of mindfulness.* Berkeley, CA: Parallax Press.

The author is a Buddhist monk who was exiled from his home country for peace activism during the Vietnam War. This text, one of many he has published that address meditative practice, includes his translations of ancient Buddhist scriptures. These particular teachings of Buddha, called sutra in Sanskrit, describe the process of becoming mindful. Mindfulness, being fully aware, is the spiritual purpose of meditation in the Zen tradition. In addition to providing the translations from Pali, Sanskrit, and Chinese, the author includes a discussion of the sutras and various meditation exercises based on the sutras. Characteristic of Zen practice, many of the exercises are elegantly simple in design, while others focus on complex problems of human existence such as Overcoming Guilt and Fear, Observing Anger, and Healing Wounds with Awareness of Joy.

MEDITATION: GENERAL INTEREST

Norris, G. (1991). *Being home: A book of meditations.* New York: Bell Tower.

An inspirational pocket-size text of readable meditations about the common and ordinary aspects of life—making the bed, climbing stairs, opening the window, for example. The text is complemented by black and white photos of objects in the home by Greta Sibley.

This text parallels the method used by Buddhist monks to spiritualize the elements of daily life. This author has also raised the mundane duties of household tasks to a level of spiritual awareness. In perusing these slices of real life, the reader becomes acutely aware of the importance of attending to the moment. Ordinary household duties are not mindless physical activities, rather they are portrayed as the substance of our lives.

Schaef, A. W. (1990). *Meditations for women who do too much.* San Francisco: Harper & Row.

This is a purse-size book that includes a brief reading meditation for each day of the year with introductory quotations written entirely by female authors. Common themes included are releasing codependence, saying no, and stress reduction presented in the context of the modern life of women. This author captures the dilemma of women who aspire to achieve in the working world, who have family commitments, and still desire some inner peace of mind. As inferred by the title, this book speaks to the contemporary complaint that women "can't have it all." However, the flow of the content provides a balanced perspective of how women should limit expectations, their own and those others place on them, in a healthy fashion.

Appendix

B CLIP-OUT NOTES AND EXERCISES

HOW TO REFOCUS CONCENTRATION DURING MEDITATION

- Passively acknowledge the intrusion by the invading thought.
- Do not follow this thought or add to it.
- Avoid traveling with your stream of consciousness.
- Bring your mind's eye back to the original focus.
- Repeat this process as many times as is necessary.
- Take no account of how many times this occurs.
- Consider each return to the point of focus as a mark of success.
- Repeat these successes as many times as necessary.

THE BASICS OF MEDITATION

- Breathing   Deep breathing at a slow regular pace.

- Body position Assume the position most comfortable for you that will allow you to stay awake through the entire procedure.

- Concentration Center your thoughts on your breathing. Aids to concentration include soothing music or training your eyes on an inanimate object or a point of light in a darkened room.

- Start slowly   Begin with meditation periods of only 5–10 minutes and spend about half that time going through the steps to relax each body part.

BASIC BEGINNER'S EXERCISE

Basic Form

- Go slowly and allow yourself about 10–15 minutes.
- Assume your position of comfort.
- Proceed with each activity gently and without rushing.

When You Are Ready

- Take three slow, full deep breaths.
- During each inspiration, feel how the air moves inward through your nose, traveling to the lungs.
- Create a mental picture of how the air fills that space in your lungs.
- Hold that first breath, gently, for just a few seconds. Then, release your breath slowly and evenly through the mouth.
- Feel the air move slowly across your air passages, across the tongue, and out the lips.
- Feel the movement of your abdomen as your lungs fill with air and become empty again.
- Experience your breathing and do not allow thoughts and ideas to disrupt your concentration on your breath.
- Continue your breathing.
- Pay close attention to how breathing feels, how the moving air feels, and the effects breathing has on your body as a whole.
- Center yourself again in your breathing.
- You may return your concentration to your breathing at any time and thus complete the meditation.
- When you are finished, gently open your eyes.
- Gently reawaken your body with some gentle stretching exercises before rising to your feet. Make the transition out of meditation a calm and peaceful process.

INTRODUCTORY PROGRESSIVE
RELAXATION EXERCISE

When your group is prepared to begin, have them assume a comfortable position. Follow each of the instructions listed below as directed. Do not hurry or rush through them.

When the group is fully relaxed, read as follows:

- This is a special time for you, a time of meditation, a time of peace and relaxation. Softly, easily, let your eyes gently drift closed.

- Use your breathing to center yourself. Breathe deeply in and then deeply out. (pause) Slowly in, and slowly out.

- Release the thoughts and concerns of the outside world. (pause) Let your breathing be your guide for this meditation. (pause) Slowly in and slowly out. (pause) Slowly in and slowly out.

- As you breathe in, you can feel a powerful and calming energy flow into your lungs with each breath.

- As you exhale, each out-breath takes with it all your tension and fatigue. (pause) All that is left is perfect relaxation and a feeling of great peace.

- Feel that calming energy flow in like the crest of a wave with each in-breath. (pause) As certainly and calmly as it rushes in, it flows back out again in one cleansing sweep.

- Breathing in, breathing out, (pause) feel your whole body relaxing and releasing tension with every breath, (pause) releasing worry with every breath.

- Feel the gentle sensation of your clothing upon your skin. (pause) Feel the rhythmic sensation of your breathing.

- Still gently breathing in and breathing out, bring your attention to your feet. (pause) In your mind's eye, visualize the calming energy flowing in, flowing like waves on the shore.

- Feel that energy surging through your body to your feet and back out again, taking with it all tension and stress.

- *Breathing in and breathing out, let your attention move upward to your legs. (pause) Feel the weight of your legs. (pause) Feel how your breathing energizes your legs, drawing out any tension or fatigue.

- *The waves of energy from your in-breathing continue to rush down through your legs and feet.

- *The warm yet tranquil waves wash away all tension. (pause) Each breath brings new refreshment, each wave becomes a surge of peaceful warm energy.

- It is now time to end the exercise. You may now return your concentration to your breathing. (pause) You may now slowly open your eyes.

NOTE: To progressively relax the entire body repeat the preceding instructions marked with an asterisk (*) and insert the names of other parts of the body (arms and hands, torso and back, head and neck). Move the focus of relaxation from the feet toward the head. Depending on how long the exercise is planned to be, additional time can be used for meditating on breathing alone.

COUNTING THE BREATH

When You Are Ready

- In your mind's eye, visualize the number one at some distance from your body.

- When you slowly inhale, visualize this number being sucked into your lungs with the air you breathe.

- Picture the number one entering your nose, passing through your upper airways, down into your lungs, and mixing with the air down there.

- Watch this number being exhaled back through your airways and out through your lips. Waiting there before you for your second breath is the number two.

- Imagine that this number becomes your second breath and travels the path of your breathing.

- Give each breath its own identity. Do not allow yourself to slur the details of how each breath travels into your lungs and out again.

- Occupy your mind with the details of each aspect of each respiratory event.

- As wandering thoughts intrude on your concentration, recognize them and allow them to pass from consciousness.

- Return your concentration to your breathing whenever you are ready to finish and thus complete the meditation.

NOTE: In the counting method, each breath is counted from one to ten. If you find your mind wandering at any point in counting, stop and start over with the number one again. Whenever your counting concentration is broken, gently return to the number one and start over again.

SENSING THE BREATH

When You Are Ready

- Take on each breath as you would take a sip of cool water on a thirsty day.

- From the first breath, feel the air as it passes through your nose. Is it cool or is it warm?

- Can you feel its fluid movement over the soft structures at the back of the throat? (pause) Notice the difference in how the air feels moving inward compared to moving outward.

- As you fill your lungs, feel the outward movement of the chest and abdomen. Do your clothes move ever so slightly against your skin?

- Sense the slight movement of your chest against your upper arms and your clothing.

- Notice how your heart rate increases slightly with each inward breath and slows again with each exhale.

- Allow yourself a moment to appreciate the perfection of the warm sensations of feeling relaxed and calm.

- Ever so gently, release this breath, allowing it to slowly flow back out. Savor each element of the experience without rushing.

- Consider each breath as a perfect refreshing moment. Although each one is perfect, there is no limit on how many perfect moments or perfect breaths we are each allowed.

- To complete the exercise, return your concentration to your breathing.

SLOWING THE BREATH

When You Are Ready

- Without exerting any perceptible effort, slightly increase the volume of your breath. When the volume is increased, there is a tendency to exhale more quickly. Resist this temptation. Neither should you hold your breath in the usual fashion by closing your airway.

- Make the pause between inspiration and expiration as effortless as possible. This moment is an interlude, a peaceful episode. The beating of your heart should be your only companion in that moment.

- Feel the rhythm of your breathing, the gentle in and the gentle out. Dwell on the slow and peaceful cadence.

- Follow each in-breath and each out-breath with your attention. Occasionally open yourself to the sensations from the rest of your body.

- Savor each perfect peaceful sensation. Become a sponge to the calming physical effect of sensing your breath.

- Explore the feeling of well-being it conveys; become intimate with it.

- Reach for this feeling and reconstruct it each time you contemplate your breathing, even when you are not meditating.

- Return your concentration to your breathing to complete the meditation exercise.

WALKING MEDITATION

When You Are Ready

- Stand tall and erect without moving. Allow your arms to hang relaxed from your shoulders. Take a few slow, deep breaths.

- As you begin to take your first step, slowly lift your leg and foot upward. Sense the weight of your lower leg and foot.

- Swing the foot forward, making your foot the pendulum attached to your knee. Feel the momentum of the swing on your foot and lower leg.

- Place your foot gently but firmly on the ground, taking care that you do not overextend the length of your usual gait. Notice how the foot adjusts in shape to being placed on the ground. Listen for the sound of your footstep.

- Fully place the weight of your body on this foot and leg. Take into consciousness the upright position of your body, the placement of each arm, the tilt of your head and neck.

- Continue to breathe softly and easily to avoid holding your breath at any time.

- Allow the heel of the remaining foot to lift slightly and rock upward.

- Slowly and carefully lift the remaining leg and foot, with the tip of the toes being last to leave the ground. Turn your attention to the bottom of your foot. Attend to the sensation apparent when the weight of the body is fully removed from this foot.

- Feel the arc of the pendulum of this foot in motion. Does one leg brush against the other? Can you hear your clothing rustle? Does your foot create the slightest movement of the air next to your other leg?

- As you place your foot ahead of the other, pay attention

to how your balance changes from side to side. Feel the movement of your lower arms and hands against the outer portion of your upper legs.

- Listen to the sounds created by your clothing and movement.

- Return your attention now to your other foot and leg. Continue to work through each separate sensation and movement of walking and turning.

- Return your concentration to your breathing at any point in the process and thus complete the meditation.

NOTES: Try to maintain an even pace throughout the exercise to aid in concentration. You may also add counting from one to ten to the walking meditation exercise. This is helpful to crowd out intrusive thoughts.

THE TEA CEREMONY

When You Are Ready

- Before beginning, take several deep and slow breaths.

- Gently pick up your empty tea kettle with your hand. Notice if the handle is cool or warm to your touch. Feel the weight of the kettle in your hand.

- Gently and easily turn to the water faucet. Place your hand on the handle while noting its temperature and texture.

- Place the kettle under the water spout and turn the water on at a moderate flow rate.

- Listen to the voice of the water falling into the kettle's empty interior. Notice how the sound changes as the water level rises.

- Watch the thousands of swarming bubbles flowing around the plunging flow of water into the kettle.

- When the kettle is filled, turn off the water and lift the kettle. Feel how much heavier the kettle is now than it was before.

- Turn back to the stove and place the kettle on the burner. Note the sensation of each footstep and the sound of your movements.

- Place your hand on the knob that lights and adjusts the heat. Is the surface of the knob smooth or rough, warm or cool?

- Turn on the heat under the kettle, listening for the sound made by the switch. Listen for the sound of the flame or the tapping noises of the heating element.

- Carefully attend to your breathing as the water heats. Watch for the tiny steam vapors that waft over the surface of the water before it boils and that emanate from the sides of the kettle.

- Listen for the tiniest bubbles that germinate from the sides of the kettle and rise to the water's surface. Marvel at their number and their energy while breathing softly in and out.

- To prepare for tea, open the cupboard, being mindful of reaching and stretching with your arms. Take your favorite tea cup in hand. Feel its weight and the smooth, round surface.

- Place it on the counter before you. Peer into its hollow, shiny center. Mentally rest there for a moment.

- Take in hand the tiny envelope of tea. It is so light and delicate. Carefully lift the flap of its wrapper. Listen for the faint but abrupt sounds of the paper wrapper as you peel back the flap. Under the flap, you see a colored tab on the end of a string. Notice the shape, color, and texture of the paper tab crossed at an angle with a fine metal staple to hold the string.

- The faintest scent of the dried tea catches your attention. This delicate and pleasant scent permeates your awareness. Unhurriedly, you linger in the aroma.

- Taking the tab in your hand, pull the full length of string away from the envelope. Feel the tug when you have pulled the string taut. Listen for the sound of paper against paper as the bag of tea slides from the envelope.

- Watch the tiny bag swing out and away from the envelope. See how it swings back again like the pendulum of a clock. With the other hand, grasp the tiny bag of tea leaves. Gently feel the crunchy contents between your fingers.

- Lift the bag over the opening of the tea cup. Slowly lower the bag to rest in its waiting bowl. Rest your gaze and your concentration there in the cup with the tea bag.

- Turn your gaze again to the boiling kettle. Listen to the rush of the agitated water while you turn off the heat. As you reach toward the handle of the kettle, notice how warm the air becomes as your hand nears it.

- Slowly grasp the kettle's handle while avoiding the spout steam. Firmly and carefully lift the kettle over the waiting cup.

- Catch the first aroma of steaming water rushing over the tiny bag of tea. Watch how the water swirls round and round in the cup. See how the vortex pulls the tea bag with it. Notice how the boiling water has begun to darken slightly from the tea.

- Safely place the kettle back on the stove and notice how heavy the kettle is now, one cup lighter.

- Return your attention to the cup of brewing tea. After only moments, the color of the water has changed even more. You can see the essence of the tea swirling from the surface of the tiny bag containing the tea leaves.

- Breathing in the aroma of tea, gently touch the sides of the tea cup with your fingertips. The smooth surface of the cup is gingerly warm to touch. Reside in this compelling moment, pulled between desiring the first sip and fearing the heat.

- In a smooth, unhurried motion, lift the cup to your lips. Your breath disturbs and pulls at the streaks of steam that rise from the cup. With great care, gently direct your breath and blow it over the tea, causing ripples on its surface.

- Purse your mouth and take in the smallest sip of tea.

- Return your concentration to your breathing now or at any time to complete the meditation.

NOTE: The meditation exercise described here ends with the first sip of tea because the focus of the exercise is the preparation of the tea, not the drinking of it. The activity is the meditation.

BUBBLES MEDITATION

When You Are Ready

- Picture yourself sitting comfortably at the bottom of a cool, clear lake. (pause) You feel relaxed and very fluid like the water surrounding you.

- Breathe deeply and calmly several times to allow yourself to fully relax.

- In this meditative state, observe how extraneous thoughts intrude on your consciousness.

- Recognize these thoughts as intruders. (pause) Calmly and gently watch as one of these intrusive thoughts becomes encapsulated in a silvery bubble of air. (pause) The thought takes shape and immediately begins its peaceful ascent to the surface.

- Although your eyes are closed and the picture is only in your mind, every detail is sharp and clear. (pause) Notice how the bubble constantly and gently changes shape as it moves through the water. See how it weaves and darts upward at a slow and predictable pace.

- With full attention, watch this thought travel the long distance to the water's surface.

- The bubble has finally reached the top. (pause) You can even see the concentric ripples it causes on the surface of this cool, clear lake above you.

- Every thought that trespasses your concentration is immediately reshaped into a silvery bubble. (pause) At the instant of its transformation, it begins the wafting trip to the surface.

- Here is another intruder. (pause) How quickly it is snatched into the form of an air bubble. (pause) It moves quickly up and away.

- Proceed with the identification and entrapment of the intruding thoughts. Watch them become separate from you and make their way to the surface above you.

- Whenever you are ready, return your concentration to your breathing and complete the meditation.

BASKING IN THE LIGHT MEDITATION

When You Are Ready

- With your eyes closed, assume a comfortable position, preferably a sitting position.

- Center yourself in your breathing. (pause) Follow each breath slowly in and slowly out. (pause) Dwell in each moment and in each in-breath and each out-breath.

- In your consciousness, visualize yourself in a dark and empty space. (pause) Allow yourself to feel perfectly relaxed and comfortable in this space and at this moment.

- Directly above and in front of you, you see a tiny twinkling of light that pierces the darkness.

- This tiny ray of light now doubles in size but shines only on you. All else is shadowed in darkness.

- This clear, bright beam again doubles in size as you begin to feel its warmth on your face and forehead. (pause) Ever so slightly, tilt your head back to catch more of its warmth on your face.

- The warmth of this light seems to flow in waves across your upper body. (pause) You begin to feel the light relax the muscles of your face while the slightest hint of a smile creeps across your lips.

- The column of light gently warms your shoulders and your arms. (pause) You turn the palms of your hands upwards to catch the warmth of the light.

- Your hands and your fingers begin to feel warm and very relaxed. (pause) You can feel the tingle of your circulation in your hands and fingers stimulated by the light.

- You peacefully and gently dwell in this circle of light. (pause) The waves of gentle relaxation continue to wash down your body from your face and head, (pause) now to your shoulders, (pause) now to your upper arms, (pause) and now all the way to your hands and fingers.

- Whenever you are ready to complete the meditation simply return your concentration to your breathing.

MEDITATION ON COMPASSION

When You Are Ready

- Make yourself comfortable in whatever position suits you best to remain attentive throughout the exercise. (pause) Go slowly through each step of the relaxation process and avoid rushing yourself.

- Center yourself by taking great care to concentrate on your breathing. (pause) Experience the physical sensations of each breath. (pause) Drink in each breath, slowly in and slowly out.

- While in this deep, relaxed state, think about all of the patients and families you have encountered over your time in nursing, no matter how short.

- Think back and remember, did you ever have a patient or family member that made you angry? (pause) What did she do to make you angry? (pause) What did you do in return? (pause) How has this experience changed the way you treat your patients and their families now?

- Did a patient or a family member ever physically hurt you? (pause) What did he do to injure you? (pause) What did you do in return? (pause) How has this experience changed the way you treat your patients and their families now?

- Did a patient or family member ever hurt your feelings? (pause) What did she do to hurt your feelings? (pause) What did you do in return? (pause) How has this experience changed the way you treat your patients and their families now?

- Have you ever made one of your patients angry? (pause) Have you ever caused one of your patients undue pain or discomfort? (pause) Have you ever caused hurt feelings in one of your patients? (pause) How have these experiences changed the way you treat your patients and their families now?

- Did you ever have a patient that reminded you of your-self, that you personally identified with? (pause) What was it about him that made you personally identify with him?

- Mentally change places with this person for just one second. (pause) How does this make you feel about this person? (pause) What makes him angry or sad or hurts his feelings? (pause) What makes you angry or sad or hurts your feelings?

- What will you do differently to better care for your patients and their families?

MANTRA MEDITATION

- Take all the time you need to become fully relaxed.
- Center yourself in your breathing. Come back to it at any time to recenter yourself during the meditation period.
- Softly and gently repeat the mantra to yourself. Use your mantra with your breathing to set up a smooth and easy rhythm.
- Concentrate on your mantra and the cycles of repetition. If outside thoughts intrude, refocus yourself on your breathing and then on your mantra.
- When you have completed your meditation period, return to your breathing and thus complete your meditation exercise.

GUIDED MEDITATION: RELEASING

When You Are Ready

- Assume a comfortsble position that will also allow atten-tiveness throughout the exercise. (pause) Go slowly through the process and avoid rushing any step.

- Work through the steps to relax the body systematically and completely using your breathing.

- Center yourself in your breathing. (pause) Experience your body and your breathing in the present moment. (pause) Allow yourself to drift on each breath you take. Slowly in and slowly out, thoroughly relaxed.

- While in this deep, relaxed state, visualize a natural pool of clear, blue water surrounded by lush green ferns and almost overgrown with fern-like trees.

- Looking down into the water, you can even see the small pebbles lying deep below the water. (pause) The water is peaceful and quiet.

- There are the tiniest ripples on the surface. These tiny waves move silently toward the far edge just out of sight.

- Now you can barely hear the sound of the tiny ripples flowing out of the pool through the trees beyond.

- A leaf from an overhanging tree floats gently onto the surface of the water almost within your reach. (pause)

- The soft, green leaf lingers there, floating on the mir-rored surface. It does not sink, but drifts like a fragile boat.

- Almost imperceptibly, the leaf begins to glide uncer-tainly toward the far side of the pool. You admire how gently and peacefully the leaf makes its way to the tiny waterfall on the far side.

- Suddenly, the leaf disappears over the edge out of sight. You cannot see the leaf, but again you hear the ripple of flowing water. (pause)

- You breathe in the peace and quiet, resting quietly in its beauty.

- In this calm and relaxed state, you mentally reach into your pocket and take out a small piece of paper and a small pencil.

- You have had something on your mind recently that has worried you greatly. You are here at the water's edge because you are ready to release this worry from your consciousness.

- In a word or two, you write the nature of this problem on the small slip of paper. (pause)

- Having done so, you slowly put the pencil back in your pocket and hold the piece of paper at arm's length over the pool of silent water.

- Breathing deeply, you affirm to yourself that the out-come of this worry or problem will be for the better. In doing so, you also forgive yourself for any role you have played in the problem and forgive any other person for her role in the problem.

- You also release any anger or frustration over this prob-lem as you prepare to release this problem from your consciousness and the paper from your grip. Like a slow-motion film, you clearly see your fingers open wide and the tiny slip of paper dip and dive down out of your grip.

- The note looks like it barely touches the water and cir-cles there peacefully for a moment. (pause)

- The words you wrote on the paper are already wet as the paper takes the route of the leaf to the pool's far edge.

- You breathe deeply and calmly, watching this problem detach itself from you and move away. You also detach yourself from the emotions surrounding this problem. There is no more struggle, no more frustration.

- Suddenly the note is gone, having slipped out of the pool down behind the trees.

- Again you can barely hear the murmur of softly falling water.

- The relief from the burden is evident on your face. You carry a smile of affection and peace, a gentle smile.

- You breathe deeply and remind yourself that this peaceful place is always here for you. You can return at will and bring other problems to the water's edge. (pause) The water is there for your refreshment.

- When you are ready to finish, return your concentration to your breathing and thus complete the meditation.

GUIDED MEDITATION: ON PAIN

When You Are Ready

- Assume a comfortable position that will also allow attentiveness throughout the exercise. (pause) Go slowly through the process and avoid rushing any step.

- Work through the steps to relax the body systematically and completely using your breathing.

- Center yourself in your breathing. (pause) Experience your body and your breathing in the present moment, both the painful sensations and the warm pleasant ones. (pause)

- Turn your consciousness to the pain. (pause) What are the sensations that make up the pain message? (pause) Is the pain message steady or intermittent? (pause) What is the nature of the pain?

- What is the pain message? (pause) Are there emotions tied to the pain message? (pause) Recognize those messages, the anger, fear, or anxiety.

- Breathe with the sensations of the pain message. (pause) Become mindful of the physical and emotional aspects of this sensation called pain. (pause)

- Visualize your breath moving through the body part where the pain arises. (pause) Visualize each calm and peaceful breath flowing through the pain. (pause)

- Recognize that the pain sensation is only a sensation and nothing else. (pause) The pain is not part of your identity and you do not own this pain. (pause) You are merely experiencing pain at this time.

- Accept the pain as an aspect of this present moment. (pause) Do not react to the pain or judge it.

- Distance yourself from the sensations of the pain experience. (pause) Release any emotional interpretations you have about your pain. (pause)

- Dwell in the moment of the experience. (pause) Just be present here and now.

- Use your breathing to massage and destress the pain experience.

- Return your concentration to your breathing at any time and thus complete the meditation.

GUIDED MEDITATION: WORKING THROUGH GRIEF

When You Are Ready

- Assume a comfortable position that will also allow you to be attentive, yet relaxed, throughout this exercise.

- Center yourself in your breathing. (pause) Experience the sensations of your body and your breathing in the present moment. With each in-breath and each out-breath, let yourself experience each pleasant and peaceful sensation.

- Focus totally on your breathing. (pause) There is no past moment or future moments, only the present moment. (pause) Dwell in the sensations of how you feel right now, so calm and peaceful.

- In your mind's eye, see yourself in a warm, sunlit room where time cannot intrude. You are calm and everything is at peace. (pause) As you breathe deeply, you feel a great sense of well-being. (pause) Experience every in-breath and every out-breath as a now experience.

- While resting in this timeless room, full of peace and warmth, thoughts of a special person come to mind. This special person is no longer with you now in the physical sense, because he has passed on. (pause) However, in your mind, you bring all of your good thoughts and favorite memories of this special person into this warm and peaceful room with you.

- In your mind's eye, see yourself and this special person sitting together, quietly enjoying the company of each other in this wonderful place. (pause) You have no need for words. You are both very calm and everything is at peace. (pause) Again when you breathe deeply, you both feel a great sense of well-being from being here together in the endless present moment. (long pause)

- While you abide together in this quiet place, there is no pain or suffering permitted. (pause) There is only peace and calm. (pause) As you abide together in this quiet place, there is no fear or grief. (pause) There is only peace and love. (long pause)

- You dwell in this peaceful place together until you and your special person are completely saturated with the company of each other. (long pause)

- Having shared this timeless time with your special person in your consciousness, remember that this place always exists for you to recall this special person.

- When you are satisfied, you can bring your consciousness back to your breathing. Even in doing so, you retain that feeling of warmth and comfort from remembering your special person. Let this feeling linger. Hold on to it. Make it last.

GUIDED MEDITATION: FORGIVENESS

When You Are Ready

- Assume a comfortable position that will also permit you to be attentive throughout the exercise. (pause) Go slowly and avoid rushing any step.

- Center yourself in your breathing. (pause) Experience your body and your breathing in the present moment in complete relaxation.

- When you are fully centered, you are completely safe and secure. (pause) You are fully insulated from the outside world, yet perfectly free and safe.

- While in this safe and secure place, envision the person you love most in the universe. This person can be anyone you love the most, living or dead. In your mind's eye, envision your loved one healthy and happy and whole.

- Now take a minute to smile to yourself and enjoy the mental presence of your loved one. (pause) Remember all of the good things about this person and the love you feel for her. (pause) Hold those good thoughts.

- Do you remember the good times laughing and talking with this person? Does it make you smile again? Do you remember the sound of her voice, her funny expressions? (pause) Hold those good feelings.

- Right now, experience how your body feels when you think about this person you love the most in the universe. (pause) Do you feel warm and happy? Can you feel the smile on your face? (pause) Feel on the inside what you are feeling on the outside.

- With this vision of your loved one in your mind's eye, ask yourself a question. What if something very bad happened because this person made a bad decision or made a mistake? Would you forgive her for what happened? (pause) Of course, you would forgive the person you love most in the universe. She deserves your love and forgiveness, doesn't she?

- What does that forgiveness feel like to your body? (pause) How does forgiveness feel inside you? (pause) Think about your loved one and experience this feeling of forgiving. (pause) In the silence of your heart, speak words of loving forgiveness to your loved one.

- Forgiveness erases the pain and distress. (pause) Afterwards, there is no more guilt to forgive.

- Center yourself again in your breathing. (pause) Experience again this safe and secure space in your consciousness.

- Now turn your conscious focus to yourself. In your own heart, answer this question: Have you ever felt guilty because something bad happened to you, or you made a bad decision, or you made a mistake? (pause) How does this guilt feel to your body?

- Although you may have carried this guilt with you for a long time, think how quickly you were ready to forgive the person you loved most in the universe. (pause) In your mind's eye, mentally see yourself as that person you love most in the universe. Just as you did before, go through the experience of feeling forgiveness and being forgiven.

- In the silence of your heart, speak words of loving forgiveness to yourself. (pause) What does that forgiveness feel like to your body? (pause) How does forgiveness feel inside you? (pause) Think about yourself and experience this feeling of forgiving and forgiveness.

- Forgiveness erases the guilt and the pain and the distress. (pause) Afterwards, there is no more guilt to forgive. You are forgiven. You are completely forgiven. Feel the forgiveness.

- Center yourself again in your breathing. (pause) Experience again this safe and secure place in your consciousness. (pause) Remember, you can return to this place at any time you desire. This place is a well of peace and forgiveness. Come and drink from it any time you desire.

- You may return your concentration to your breathing at any time and thus complete the meditation.

I N D E X